New Frontiers for the Treatment of Keratoconus

César Carriazo · María José Cosentino
Editors

New Frontiers for the Treatment of Keratoconus

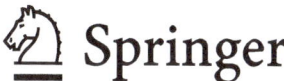 Springer

Editors
César Carriazo
University Del Norte
Barranquilla, Atlantico
Colombia

María José Cosentino
University of Buenos Aires
Buenos Aires
Argentina

ISBN 978-3-030-66142-7   ISBN 978-3-030-66143-4   (eBook)
https://doi.org/10.1007/978-3-030-66143-4

This Springer imprint is published by the registered company Springer Nature Switzerland AG
The registered company address is: Gewerbestrasse 11, 6330 Cham, Switzerland

Foreword

With the new imaging modalities, keratoconus is being diagnosed more frequently at earlier stages than in the past; it is clear now that the incidence and prevalence of keratoconus, may have been underestimated.

There have been reports of this disorder since more than a century, but until 1986 the only possible treatment was contact lenses and in advanced cases, corneal transplantation.

Since then, a huge advance in technological developments has been introduced and a number of treatment options are in our hands. These advances and treatment modalities range from: corneal ring segments to flatten the anterior 5.0 or 6.0 mm central corneal radius, corneal collagen cross-linking to arrest the progression of the disorder, phakic lenses, and corneal refractive surgery to improve visual acuity as well as also a combination of these procedures. Corneal grafts are the last resource, Pre-Descemet lamellar grafts being the first option nowadays.

This book contains the knowledge and experience of a group of important people who have done scientific research in the field of keratoconus, have developed the diagnostic tools that have improved its early detection, and have developed and perfected the treatment modalities that we have in our arsenal today.

César Carriazo and María José Cosentino, creative ophthalmic surgeons and editors of this book, are presenting to us a new surgical technique for keratoconus treatment, founded on ideas and experiences of their professors, but with a different reasoning. After deep biomechanical, histopathological, and computer simulation studies and with the precision of actual laser technologies, are presenting a different approach to reconstruct the shape of the anterior corneal surface in keratoconus.

As Drs. Carriazo and Cosentino suggest in this book, until another valid alternative appears in the near future, we can count on the corneal remodeling technique as an efficient tool for the refractive treatment of keratoconus. This implies being in front of a therapeutic aid with a high impact on global public health.

The technique is under development, and there are many questions that are yet to be resolved. There will be controversies, but as Szent Györgyi said, *"Discovery must be, by definition, at variance with existing knowledge."*

Carmen Barraquer Coll
Instituto Barraquer de América
Bogotá, Colombia

Preface

Eighteen months ago, while we were at a symposium on keratoconus, the seed of this book emerged. We realized two important things: the first referred to how far the diagnostic and therapeutic management of this pathology had advanced; the second was related to a critical view of certain therapeutic alternatives. In the lectures or courses that we give, it is common to hear us say that doctors must make analysis of the medical tools they have as objective as possible.

Performing a procedure because everyone does it, or because it is the only alternative, can get us into a false situation, without the ability to discern what is best for our patients.

A few years ago, the predictability we obtained with keratoconus treatments was so poor that we used the word "orthopedic" when referring to them, so as not to compromise with the patient's refractive result. Today, the therapeutic resource that we have allows us to offer our patients a refractive visual prognosis, never the same as those obtained in healthy patients, but with the peace of mind of improving vision with a high degree of satisfaction in its result, both in quantity and visual quality.

The decision to make this book implied the elaboration of an updated scientific material, written by distinguished collaborators from a wide variety of countries and outstanding worldwide participation, true references that we chose for their indisputable merits.

The result of more than a year of painstaking work is compiled in this book, which aims to direct our gaze – if the phrase fits! – specifically towards those current tools with which we have to diagnose and treat keratoconus. This means that we have focused only on those elements that currently coexist in our practice and that will definitely have a space in the future – at least immediate – of anterior segment ophthalmology.

We have also given an important space to videos that allow us to dynamically illustrate the contents of each chapter.

We would truly like to thank the main support of our family who resign themselves to spend their time with us, understanding our passion for knowledge, scientific development and innovations. Likewise, we appreciate the collaboration of all participating authors and colleagues who encouraged us in entrepreneurship. We believe that we have met the proposed challenge: a very specific compilation aimed at updating the knowledge about an entity that definitely has a space of impact on global public health.

Barranquilla, Colombia   César Carriazo
Buenos Aires, Argentina   María José Cosentino

Contents

Panorama of the Treatment of Keratoconus in 2020   1
César Carriazo and María José Cosentino

Corneal Biomechanics and Integrated Parameters for Keratoconus
Diagnosis   7
Marcella Q. Salomão, Ana Luisa Hofling- Lima, Joana Mello,
Nelson Batista Sena Jr., and Renato Ambrósio Jr.

Corneal Topography, Corneal Tomography, and Epithelial
Maps in Keratoconus 27
Dan Z. Reinstein, Timothy J. Archer, Ryan S. Vida,
Ronald H. Silverman, and Raksha Urs

Histopathological Findings in Keratoconus 49
Sabrina Bergeron, Bruno F. Fernandes, Patrick Logan, and
Miguel N. Burnier Jr.

Customized Corneal Cross-Linking 55
Theo G. Seiler

An Essential Guide to Treat Primary Ectasia with
Intracorneal Segments 61
Roberto Gustavo Albertazzi

Phakic Intraocular Lens in Keratoconus 83
Alaa Eldanasoury, Sherif Tolees, and Harkaran S. Bains

Excimer Laser and Keratoconus 99
César Carriazo and María José Cosentino

Regencrative Therapies for Keratoconus 109
Jorge L. Alió del Barrio, Verónica Vargas, and Jorge L. Alió

Corneal Remodeling: A New Alternative Technique to Treat Corneal
Ectasia 123
César Carriazo and María José Cosentino

Index 139

Contributors

Roberto Gustavo Albertazzi Cornea and Refractive Surgery, Quilmes, Argentina

Jorge L. Alió Cornea, Cataract and Refractive Surgery Unit, Vissum Instituto Oftalmológico de Alicante, Alicante, Spain

Universidad Miguel Hernández, Alicante, Spain

Jorge L. Alió del Barrio Cornea, Cataract and Refractive Surgery Unit, Vissum Instituto Oftalmológico de Alicante, Alicante, Spain

Universidad Miguel Hernández, Alicante, Spain

Renato Ambrósio Jr. Instituto de Olhos Renato Ambrósio, Rio de Janeiro, Brazil

Rio de Janeiro Corneal Tomography and Biomechanics Study Group, Rio de Janeiro, Brazil

Brazilian Study Group of Artificial Intelligence and Corneal Analysis – BrAIN, Rio de Janeiro & Maceió, Brazil

Department of Ophthalmology, Federal University of São Paulo, São Paulo, Brazil

Department of Ophthalmology, Federal University the state of Rio de Janeiro (UNIRIO), Rio de Janeiro, Brazil

Timothy J. Archer London Vision Clinic, London, UK

Harkaran S. Bains Sight By Design, Edmonton, AB, Canada

Sabrina Bergeron The MUHC – McGill University Ocular Pathology & Translational Research Laboratory, Montreal, QC, Canada

Miguel N. Burnier Jr. The MUHC – McGill University Ocular Pathology & Translational Research Laboratory, Montreal, QC, Canada

César Carriazo Clínica Carriazo, Universidad del Norte, Barranquilla, Colombia

María José Cosentino Instituto de la Visión, Universidad de Buenos Aires, Buenos Aires, Argentina

Alaa Eldanasoury Department of Ophthalmology, Magrabi Hospital, Jeddah, Saudi Arabia

Bruno F. Fernandes The MUHC – McGill University Ocular Pathology & Translational Research Laboratory, Montreal, QC, Canada

Ana Luisa Hofling- Lima Department of Ophthalmology, Federal University of São Paulo, São Paulo, Brazil

Patrick Logan The MUHC – McGill University Ocular Pathology & Translational Research Laboratory, Montreal, QC, Canada

Joana Mello Rio de Janeiro Corneal Tomography and Biomechanics Study Group, Rio de Janeiro, Brazil

Dan Z. Reinstein London Vision Clinic, London, UK

Columbia University Medical Center, New York, NY, USA

Sorbonne Université, Paris, France

School of Biomedical Sciences, University of Ulster, Coleraine, UK

Marcella Q. Salomão Instituto de Olhos Renato Ambrósio, Rio de Janeiro, Brazil

Rio de Janeiro Corneal Tomography and Biomechanics Study Group, Rio de Janeiro, Brazil

Brazilian Study Group of Artificial Intelligence and Corneal Analysis – BrAIN, Rio de Janeiro & Maceió, Brazil

Department of Ophthalmology, Federal University of São Paulo, São Paulo, Brazil

Instituto Benjamin Constant, Rio de Janeiro, Brazil

Theo G. Seiler Universitätsklinik für Augenheilkunde, Inselspital Bern, Bern, Switzerland

Wellman Center for Photomedicine – Massachusetts General Hospital, Harvard Medical School, Boston, MA, USA

Institut für Refraktive und Ophthalmo-Chirurgie (IROC), Zürich, Switzerland

Nelson Batista Sena Jr. Rio de Janeiro Corneal Tomography and Biomechanics Study Group, Rio de Janeiro, Brazil

Department of Ophthalmology, Federal University the state of Rio de Janeiro (UNIRIO), Rio de Janeiro, Brazil

Ronald H. Silverman Columbia University Medical Center, New York, NY, USA

Sherif Tolees Department of Ophthalmology, Magrabi Hospital, Jeddah, Saudi Arabia

Raksha Urs Columbia University Medical Center, New York, NY, USA

Verónica Vargas Innovation and Investigation Department, Vissum Instituto Oftalmológico de Alicante, Alicante, Spain

Ryan S. Vida London Vision Clinic, London, UK

Panorama of the Treatment of Keratoconus in 2020

César Carriazo and María José Cosentino

Keratoconus has always been a challenge both in its early diagnosis and integral treatment. When we began this book project, we considered making an updated panorama of the diagnosis and treatment of the keratoconus. We believe the keratoconus has been and still remains one of the pathologies whose treatment has been benefited most over the last two decades.

Beginning with the diagnosis, we have made greater in the early detection helped by the new keratoconus indices, among which we can highlight Belin-Ambrosio ones. We have been also helped by the improvement and new technologies which have contributed to the early detection of such disease. In this book, we have included a handful of chapters related to the diagnosis of keratoconus. Looking forward, we believe the gene therapy will not only be the future but it will intervene in the diagnosis and treatment of the disease as well [1, 2].

There is no doubt the corneal crosslinking becomes an important procedure when it comes to both stopping the progression of the *novo keratoconus* and being used in personalized refractive treatments in an adjunct way (Fig. 1). As a results, having a more stable cornea by using crosslinking has allowed us to correct these patients in a refractive way to improve their visual quality, and in most cases, we obtained the non-use of contact lenses or glasses. We have been given the opportunity to fine-tune the target of the treatments to be able to correct refractive defects [3].

It is important to consider the inflammatory component as the essential basis for the keratoconus. This has opened a wide range of possibilities of understanding its clinical ongoing process and performing different, anticipatory and more appropriate treatments avoiding advanced stages of the disease. Patients with advanced stages prevent us from using more rigid chances aimed at therapeutic strategies, and as a consequence, we are only able to perform a keratoplasty.

C. Carriazo
Clínica Carriazo, Universidad del Norte, Barranquilla, Colombia

M. J. Cosentino (✉)
Instituto de la Vision, Universidad de Buenos Aires, Buenos Aires, Argentina

© Springer Nature Switzerland AG 2021
C. Carriazo, M. J. Cosentino (eds.), *New Frontiers for the Treatment of Keratoconus*, https://doi.org/10.1007/978-3-030-66143-4_1

Fig. 1 Corneal
crosslinking

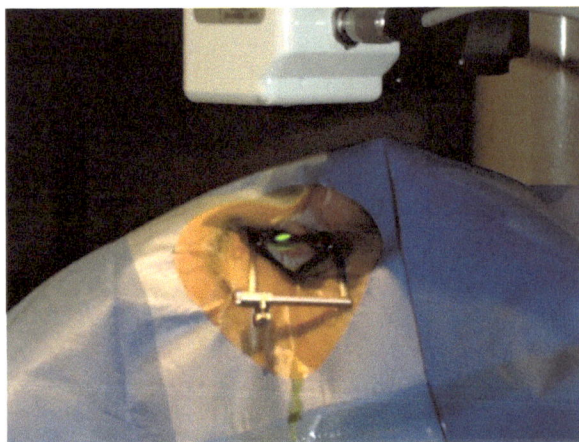

Fig. 2 Intracorneal rings

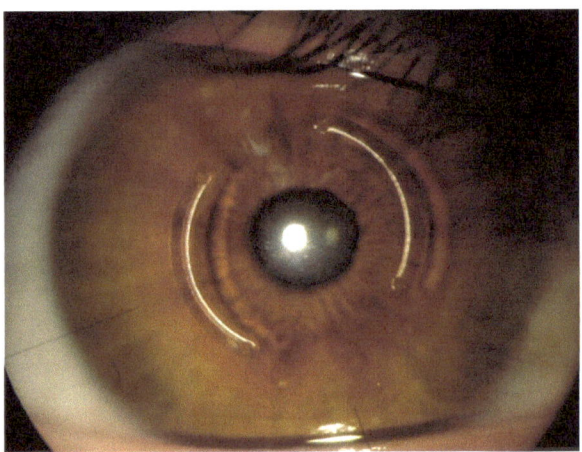

The intracorneal ring implantation has also been an alternative to correct irregular astigmatism, which is an unfortunate characteristic of the keratoconus (Fig. 2) [4, 5]. Likewise, we found the great alternative to compensate the ametropia of this type of patients either in a refractive way by means of phakic lens implantation or with the use of excimer laser by performing a photorefractive surgery. In chapters 7 and 8, the obtained results and our remarks on the best indications are shown. The use of excimer laser in patients with keratoconus is limited to a very specific segment of patients, and unfortunately the use of such laser cannot be broadly applied because it works in the corneal plane, which is the visibly affected tissue in the keratoconus [6, 7]. However, the phakic lens implantation allows correcting high ametropies, which often occur in patients with keratoconus, with really promising results (Fig. 3) [8, 9, 10]. Once these chapters have been read, we have no doubts that our readers will find the necessary grounds to count on both tools to correct these patients in a refractive way.

Fig. 3 Posterior chamber phakic intraocular lens

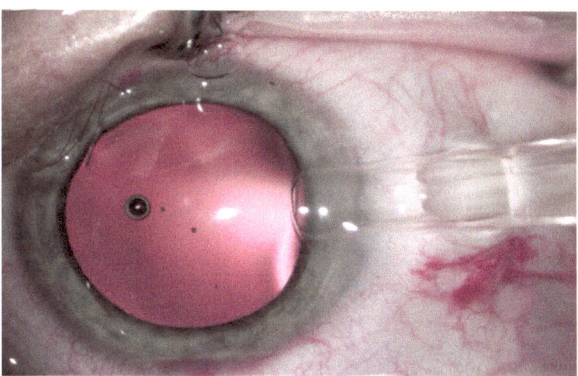

In the treatment options, we will observe that each treatment has a different biomechanical behaviour. The corneal flattening of crosslinking is due to the contraction of the stromal lamellae. This allows the stroma to become more rigid, and in many cases, a slight flattening is produced. The corneal flattening obtained after corneal crosslinking is due to the contractions of the stromal lamellae.

When we talk about corneal refractive correction, especially with laser, its biomechanical behaviour obeys Dr. José Ignacio Barraquer's law of thickness, which tells us: "If we remove tissue in the periphery or add it in the centre, we bend the cornea" and, on the contrary, "If we remove tissue in the centre or add it in the periphery, we flatten the cornea". This is a way of "carving or sculpting" the anterior structure of the cornea.

However, Barraquer's studies and findings were based on healthy corneas which he planned to modify its anterior face in order to be refractive. Therefore, this thickness law does not apply to all keratoconus corneas. Unstable and/or weak corneas do not obey this law. What must be done? How do we calculate? How do we predict their behaviour? [11].

Such is the case of corneal rings, which do not respond in essence to Dr. Barraquer's law. In the case of intracorneal ring implantation, there is no corneal carving. In these cases, the cornea is not carved, the intracorneal rings produce a "tension" generated in the posterior stroma and a consequent flattening in the anterior layers of the cornea.

A great panorama is opened with the new therapeutic alternatives to treat keratoconus. We can say that they are not palliative and compensatory; they are more radical, if the term is allowed. This type of treatment, unimaginable at the end of the twentieth century, contributes to creating a cornea with coefficients closer to normal tissue. Stromal regeneration therapy has shown very good results in that way too, and we believe it will be a solid treatment alternative, which will be consolidated in the near future. This is expressed in one of our chapters [12, 13].

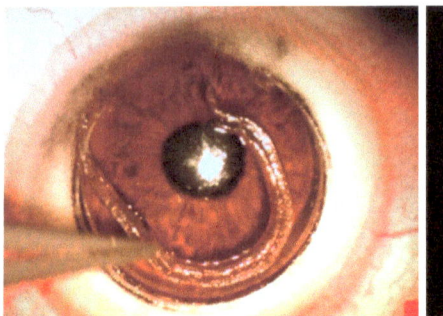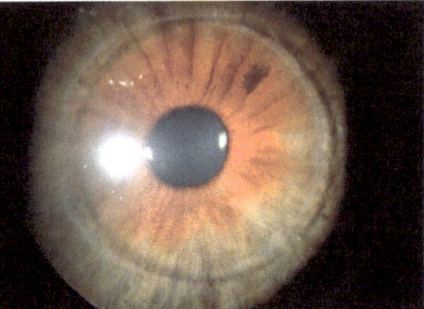

Fig. 4 Corneal remodelling

Talking about keratoconus without mentioning the concepts of corneal biome-chanics is impossible. We address new concepts on this topic that will allow us to lead the analysis from a new approach. We would like to specially highlight a new surgical alternative to treat corneal ectasia, which we have called "corneal remodel-ling" (Fig. 4) [14, 15]. This technique is a new concept that moves away from the conceptual bases of "laminar contraction", observed in corneal crosslinking; it also differs from the one observed in the Thickness Law, "carved or sculpted" and it is also far from the concept of "tense deformation", presented in intracorneal rings. Since resistance is the keyword suffered by corneas with keratoconus, with this new concept, we introduce ourselves into the generation of a new limbo, resistant, which generates a physiological corneal profile. This new concept is based on "corneal stretching", which is the essence of the procedure. The results observed encourage us to think that it becomes a valid alternative procedure between the tools of the present and the future, at least until other superior technologies appear. This new therapeutic instrument is efficient in the optical and refractive management of kera-toconus. One of its great advantages is the wide and clear optical zone, which allows optical aberrations to be modified and aims at the recovery of visual quality.

We have not included in the content of the book the alternative of performing keratoplasty, as it is our goal to give a great panorama of the immediate future that is foreseen regarding the most effective treatments for corneas with keratoconus. We believe that well-understood medicine is more corrective and less palliative.

To conclude this brief introduction, we should not take each technique as an isolated or separate treatment entity, but rather as a combinable and elastic whole, capable of being coupled in one or several procedures. One, two or more of these alternatives may be indicated simultaneously or in a deferred form. In our experi-ence, the result of the combination of therapies is usually very positive not only in the optical and biostructural treatment of keratoconus but also in the refractive improvement of our patients.

References

1. Ambrosio R Jr, Randleman JB. Screening for ectasia risk: what are we screening for and how should we screen for it? J Refract Surg (Thorofare, NJ : 1995). 2013;29:230–2.
2. Roberts CJ, Dupps WJ Jr. Biomechanics of corneal ectasia and biomechanical treatments. J Cataract Refract Surg. 2014;40:991–8.
3. Seiler TG, Fischinger I, Koller T, et al. Customized corneal cross-linking: one-year results. Am J Ophthalmol. 2016;166:14–21.
4. Colin J, et al. Correcting Keratoconus with Intracorneal Rings. J. Cataract Refract Surg. 2000;26(8):1117–22.
5. Alfonso J, Lisa C, Merayo-Lloves J, et al. Intrastromal corneal ring segment implantation in paracentral keratoconus with coincident topographic and coma axis. J Cataract Refract Surg. 2012;38:1576–82.
6. Bardan AS, Lee H, Nanavaty MA. Outcomes of simultaneous and sequential cross-linking with excimer laser. J Refract Surg. 2018 Oct 1;34(10):690–6.
7. Müller TM, Lange AP. Topography-guided PRK and crosslinking in eyes with keratoconus and post-LASIK ectasia. Klin Monbl Augenheilkd. 2017;234(4):451–4. 28192838.
8. Güell JL, Morral M, Malecaze F, Gris O, Elies D, Manero F. Collagen crosslinking and toric iris-claw phakic intraocular lens for myopic astigmatism in progressive mild to moderate keratoconus. J Cataract Refract Surg. 2012 Mar;38(3):475–84.
9. Venter J. Artisan phakic intraocular lens in patients with keratoconus. J Refract Surg. 2009 Sep;25(9):759–64.
10. Alfonso JF, Fernández-Vega L, Lisa C, Fernandes P, González-Méijome JM, Montés-Micó R. Collagen copolymer toric posterior chamber phakic intraocular lens in eyes with keratoconus. J Cataract Refract Surg. 2010 Jun;36(6):906–16.
11. Andreassen TT, Simonsen AH, Oxlund H. Biomechanical properties of keratoconus and normal corneas. Exp Eye Res. 1980;4:435–51.
12. De Miguel MP, Casaroli-Marano RP, Nieto-Nicolau N, Martínez-Conesa EM, Alió del Barrio JL, Alió JL, Fuentes S, Arnalich-Montiel F. Frontiers in regenerative medicine for cornea and ocular surface. In: Rahman AU, Anjum S, Bentham ED, editors. Frontiers in stem cell and regenerative medicine research; 2015. ISBN: 978–1–60805-995-9. Chapter 2: 92–138.
13. Yao L, Review BH. Mesenchymal stem cells and corneal reconstruction. Mol Vis. 2013;19:2237–43.
14. Carriazo C, Cosentino MJ. A novel corneal remodeling technique for the treatment of keratoconus. J Refract Surg. 2017;(12):854–56.
15. Carriazo C, Cosentino MJ. Corneal remodeling assisted by femtosecond laser: long term outcomes. J Refract Surg 2019: Surg. 2019;35(4):261–7.

Corneal Biomechanics and Integrated Parameters for Keratoconus Diagnosis

Marcella Q. Salomão, Ana Luisa Hofling- Lima, Joana Mello, Nelson Batista Sena Jr., and Renato Ambrósio Jr.

Electronic Supplementary Material The online version of this chapter (https://doi.org/10.1007/978-3-030-66143-4_2) contains supplementary material, which is available to authorized users.

M. Q. Salomão
Instituto de Olhos Renato Ambrósio, Rio de Janeiro, Brazil

Rio de Janeiro Corneal Tomography and Biomechanics Study Group, Rio de Janeiro, Brazil

Brazilian Study Group of Artificial Intelligence and Corneal Analysis – BrAIN, Rio de Janeiro & Maceió, Brazil

Department of Ophthalmology, Federal University of São Paulo, São Paulo, Brazil

Instituto Benjamin Constant, Rio de Janeiro, Brazil
e-mail: marcella@barravisioncernter.com.br

A. L. H. Lima
Department of Ophthalmology, Federal University of São Paulo, São Paulo, Brazil

J. Mello
Rio de Janeiro Corneal Tomography and Biomechanics Study Group, Rio de Janeiro, Brazil

N. B. Sena Jr.
Rio de Janeiro Corneal Tomography and Biomechanics Study Group, Rio de Janeiro, Brazil

Department of Ophthalmology, Federal University the state of Rio de Janeiro (UNIRIO), Rio de Janeiro, Brazil

R. Ambrósio Jr. (✉)
Instituto de Olhos Renato Ambrósio, Rio de Janeiro, Brazil

Rio de Janeiro Corneal Tomography and Biomechanics Study Group, Rio de Janeiro, Brazil

Brazilian Study Group of Artificial Intelligence and Corneal Analysis – BrAIN, Rio de Janeiro & Maceió, Brazil

Department of Ophthalmology, Federal University of São Paulo, São Paulo, Brazil

Department of Ophthalmology, Federal University the state of Rio de Janeiro (UNIRIO), Rio de Janeiro, Brazil

Introduction

Keratoconus (KC) and ectatic corneal diseases represent an important and current area of research. The diagnosis of corneal ectasia has improved notably over the last years because of two main reasons. First, there was a need to identify mild forms of KC and higher susceptibility to develop ectasia, since these cases present a higher risk of progressive iatrogenic corneal ectasia after laser vision correction [1–3]. Second, there were less invasive procedures recently developed, such as collagen cross-linking and intracorneal rings, that needed to be considered before a keratoplasty [4, 5].

Placido disk-based corneal topography has proved to be sensitive enough to detect ectatic disease, even in patients with unremarkable slit-lamp examination and normal visual acuity [6, 7]. Front surface corneal topography evolved into the three-dimensional reconstruction of the cornea with corneal tomography, through measurements of both anterior and posterior corneal surfaces, along with a pachymetric map. Studies have demonstrated the ability of corneal tomography to augment sensitivity to detect abnormalities in topographically normal eyes of patients with very asymmetric KC [8–14]. Furthermore, retrospective studies with patients that developed ectasia after LASIK also revealed the superiority of tomography over topography to identify susceptibility to develop such complication [15–17].

Nevertheless, there is an extensive consensus that ectasia occurs as a result of a biomechanical decompensation or weakness of the cornea [18, 19], which would initiate a cycle of pathological events resulting in secondary stromal thinning and corneal protrusion. Thus, assuming that the changes in corneal geometry denote a secondary event, characterizing the cornea beyond its shape should be essential for enhancing accuracy to identify milder forms of ectatic disease [20]. This chapter will discuss the latest developments and current status of corneal biomechanics evaluation, focusing on the most recent advances of commercially available instruments.

Ocular Response Analyzer

The ocular response analyzer (ORA; Reichert Ophthalmic Instruments, Buffalo, NY) was the first commercially available instrument for biomechanical assessment [21]. ORA was designed to compensate for corneal biomechanical properties, and hence, it provides a more accurate measurement of intraocular pressure (IOP). This non-contact tonometer (NCT) applies an air jet that deforms the cornea over a 5- to 6-mm area while monitoring its response/deformation during the applanation, through an advanced electro-optical system that captures an infrared reflex from the corneal apex (3-mm zone) [21–23]. Once the measurement starts, the air pulse deforms the cornea (ingoing phase), which passes through a first applanation moment, when pressure (P1) is registered, up to a concavity configuration. The air pressure then decreases (outgoing phase), allowing the cornea to progressively return to its normal shape while passing through a second applanation moment when pressure (P2) is once more registered (Fig. 1). The software then generates two pressure-derived parameters: corneal hysteresis (CH) and corneal resistance

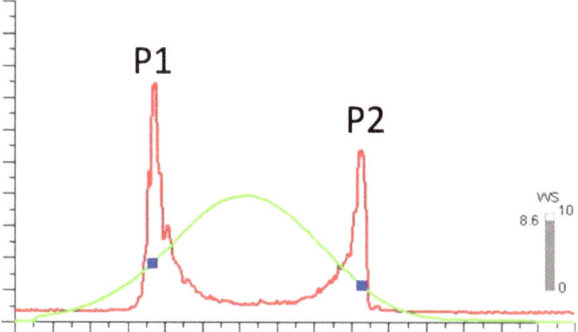

Fig. 1 Ocular response analyzer (ORA) overview display. The green curve corresponds to the air pulse and the red curve the applanation signal

factor (CRF). CII represents the difference between P1 and P2 [21–23], and CRF is derived from P1 and P2 as well, according to the formula **P1 – kP2**, where k is a constant developed by empirical evaluation of the relationship between P1, P2, and central corneal thickness.

Some disadvantages of the ORA system include high variability of measurements from the same patient, poor control of patient's head movement, and low ability of discriminating ocular diseases.

Several studies have demonstrated that CH and CRF typically present lower values and have a statistically different distribution among normal individuals versus those with KC [24], as well as in eyes following refractive procedures such as LASIK and surface ablation [25]. However, a considerable overlap in the distributions of these parameters has also been found, which limits their use for ectasia diagnosis [26, 27]. While CH and CRF have limited accuracy to distinguish between KC and normal, novel parameters derived from the waveform signal have been described, with superior results [28–32]. Furthermore, the integration of these new biomechanical data with corneal tomography has been proposed to enhance the ability to identify milder forms of ectasia. Luz and collaborators used logistic regression analysis to combine tomographic and biomechanical parameters derived from the waveform signal and found that this approach improved overall accuracy in detecting early KC (Fig. 2) [14].

Corvis ST Dynamic Scheimpflug Analyzer

The Corvis ST (Oculus, Wetzlar, Germany) is also a non-contact tonometry (NCT) system that, different from other NCT systems that monitor corneal applanation response through the reflex of an infrared beam, it uses an ultra-high-speed Scheimpflug camera with UV-free 455 nm blue light that takes 4300 frames per second to monitor corneal deformation during a consistent air-pulse application [23, 33]. Similar to what happens with the ORA, the cornea deforms inward (ingoing phase), passes through a first applanation, and continues into a concavity phase until it achieves the highest concavity (HC). The cornea then recovers and undergoes a second applanation (outgoing phase) before returning to its natural shape again.

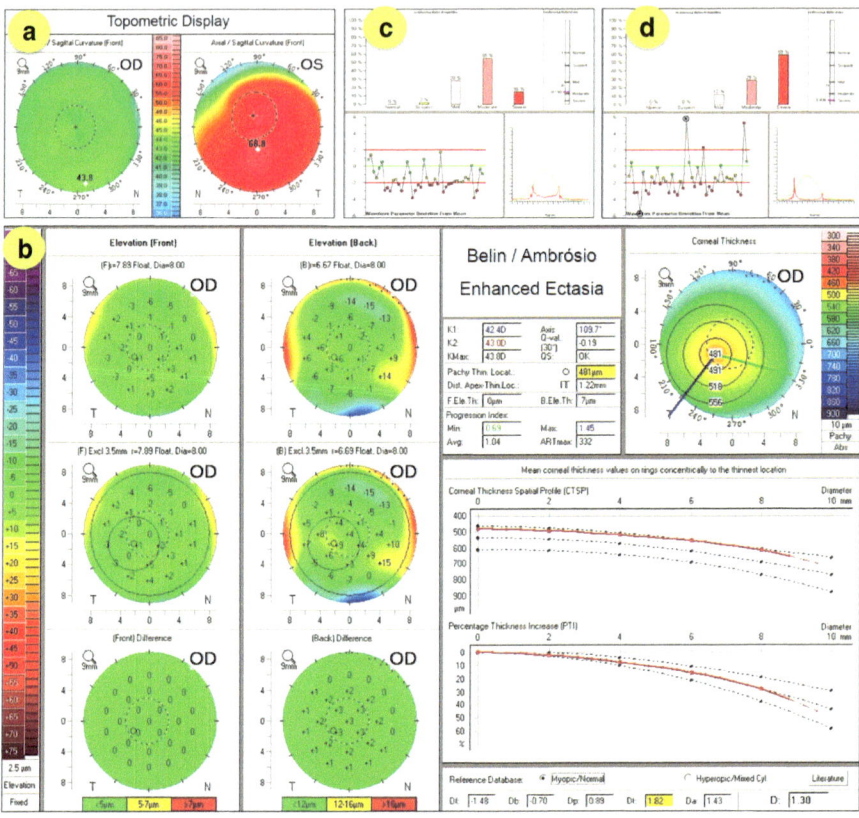

Fig. 2 Very asymmetric KC case. OD shows a relatively normal anterior curvature map from the Pentacam HR corneal tomography (Oculus Optikgeräte GmbH, Wetzlar, Germany), while OS shows advanced KC (**a**). Belin/Ambrósio enhanced ectasia display from OD demonstrates an abnormal BAD D value, higher than 1.22 (**b**). (**c**) and (**d**) represent the keratoconus match probability from OD and OS, respectively. The software integrates tomographic and biomechanical data and identifies a moderate KC match index for OD (**c**), despite a relatively normal curvature map

Different from the ORA, the maximal peak pressure of the air puff is fixed. An advantage of this device is that its measurements are less affected by ocular decentration or tear film quality.

During the whole measurement, 140 frames are taken in 32 milliseconds. The timing and corresponding pressures are monitored, and lastly, the device provides a set of corneal deformation parameters that are based on the dynamic inspection of the corneal response (Fig. 3 and Table 1) [22, 23, 33]. The deformation amplitude (DA) is detected as the highest displacement of the apex in the highest concavity (HC) moment. The radius of curvature at the highest concavity (curvature radius HC) is also recorded. Applanation lengths (AL) and corneal velocities (CVel) are documented during both ingoing and outgoing phases. Corneal thickness is also calculated through the horizontal Scheimpflug image. Figures 4, 5, 6, 7, 8, and 9 describe the Corvis parameters. IOP is calculated on the basis of the applanation pressure at the time of the first applanation, using a calibration factor (Fig. 10).

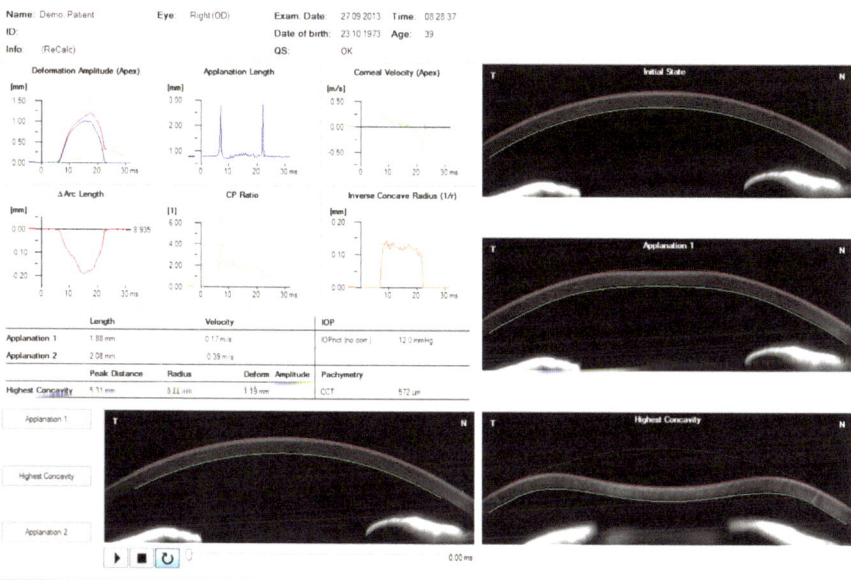

Fig. 3 Corvis ST overview display

Table 1 Corneal deformation parameters provided by the Corvis ST

1st applanation	Moment at the first applanation of the cornea during the air puff (in milliseconds). In parenthesis is the length of the applanation at this moment (in millimeters) (Fig. 4)
Highest concavity	Moment that the cornea assumes its highest concavity during the air puff (in milliseconds). In parenthesis is the length of the distance between the two peaks of the cornea at this moment (in millimeters) (Fig. 4)
2nd applanation	Moment at the second applanation of the cornea during the air puff (in milliseconds). In parenthesis is the length of the applanation at this moment (in millimeters) (Fig. 4)
Maximum deformation	Measurement (in millimeters) of the maximum cornea deformation during the air puff (Fig. 5)
Wing distance	Length of the distance between the two peaks of the cornea at this moment (in millimeters) (Fig. 7)
Maximum velocity (in)	Maximum velocity during the ingoing phase (in meters per seconds [m/s])
Maximum velocity (out)	Maximum velocity during the outgoing phase (in meters per seconds [m/s])
Curvature radius normal	Radius of curvature of the cornea in its natural state (in millimeters)
Curvature radius HC	Radius of curvature of the cornea at the time of mmHg during the air puff (in millimeters) (Fig. 6)
Corneal thickness	Measurement of corneal thickness (in millimeters) (Fig. 3)
IOP	Measurement of intraocular pressure (in millimeters of mercury [mmHg]) (Fig. 3)

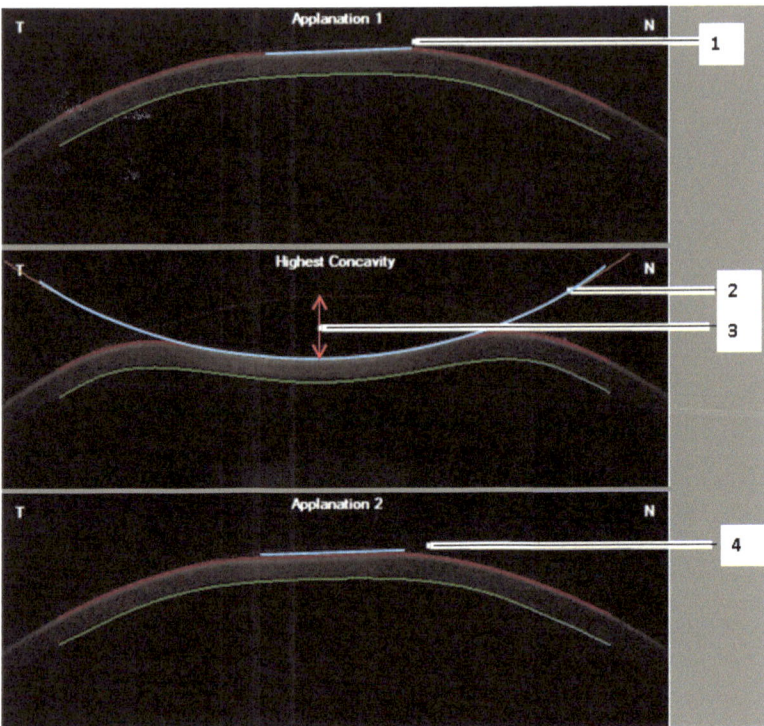

Fig. 4 Scheimpflug images representing the ingoing applanation (upper), highest concavity (middle), and outgoing applanation (lower) moments. Numbers 1 and 4 are the applanation lengths in the ingoing and outgoing phases, respectively. The applanation length is the line that describes the applanated part of the cornea, defined as having a constant slope. Number 2 represents the radius of curvature at the highest concavity or inverse concave radius. Number 3 represents the deformation amplitude at the highest concavity moment

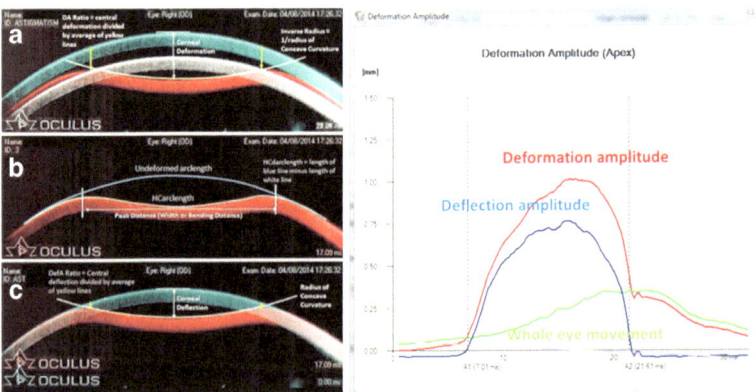

Fig. 5 Blue cornea- prior to deformation, Red cornea - maximun corneal deflection, White cornea- maximun whole eye motion. In this eye, the cornea has completely recovered. Several parameteres were developed and proven to be useful: (**a**) DA ratio - is the ratio of the central deformation divided by average of yellow lines (peripheral points located 2mm from the center). (**b**) Peak distance- is the point between the bending points of the cornea when it"s in maximum deformation. (**c**) Corneal deflection - when the periphery of these corneas is are overlaped, this gives us pure corneal motion relative to the underform state

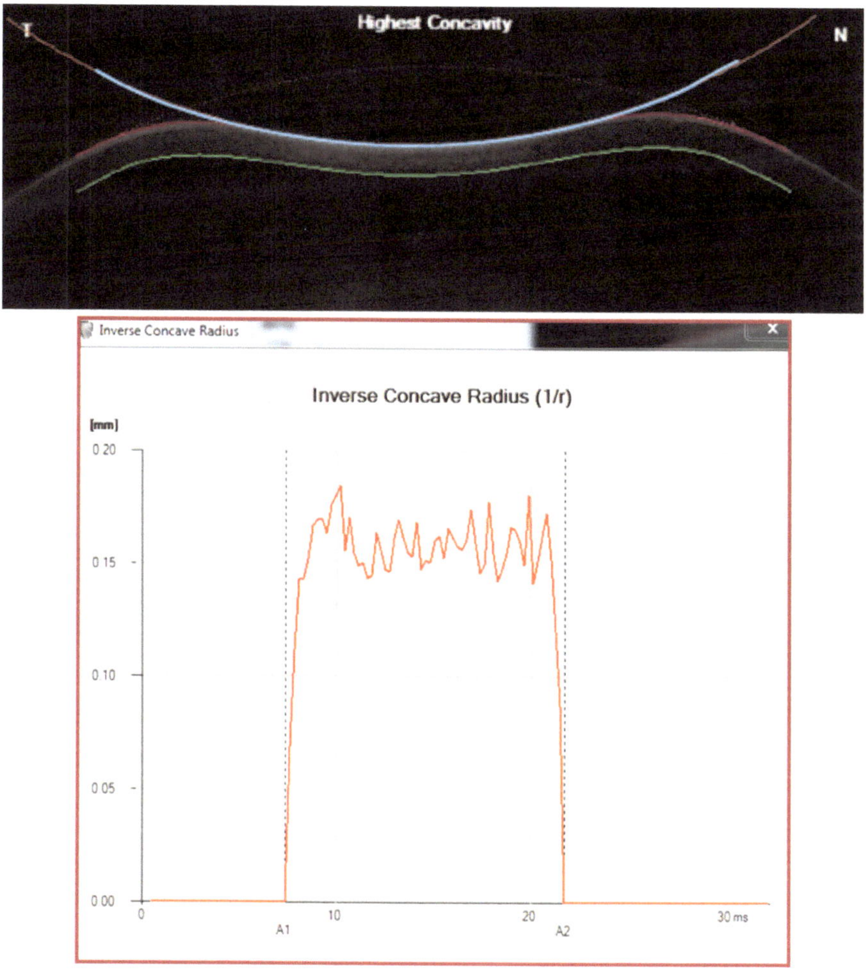

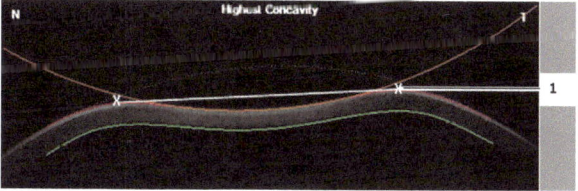

Fig. 6 Radius of curvature at the highest concavity or inverse concave radius algorithm (upper) = 1/ radius of concave curvature. The parameter has also a graphic representation, where it is plotted versus time (lower)

Fig. 7 Illustrative scheme of the peak distance parameter. The peak distance describes the distance between the two highest points of the cornea's temporal-nasal cross section at the highest concavity moment, and this is not the same as the deflection length

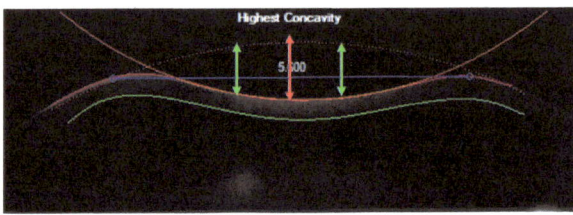

Fig. 8 Illustrative scheme of the deformation amplitude ratio between the apex and point 2 mm from the apex (DA ratio 2 mm). It describes the ratio between the deformation amplitude at the apex (red arrow) and the average deformation amplitude at the 2-mm nasal and temporal zone (green arrows)

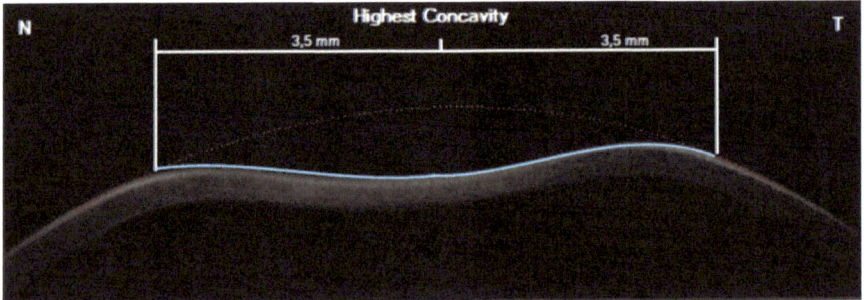

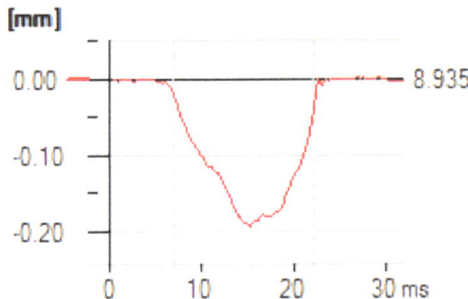

Fig. 9 Illustrative scheme of the delta arc length. It describes the change in the arc length at the highest concavity moment from the initial state, in a defined 7-mm zone. This parameter is calculated 3.5 mm from the apex to both sides in the horizontal direction

Using data from the deformation response, beyond central corneal thickness (CCT) and age, a finite element method developed by the Biomechanical Engineering Group at the University of Liverpool calculates the biomechanically compensated IOP, which is available in the Vinciguerra Screening Report [34–36].

Clinical applications to the Corvis ST system include measurement of the compensated IOP (Fig. 10), evaluating the stiffening effect of corneal cross-linking (Fig. 11), screening of refractive surgery candidates (Fig. 11), early detection of ectatic disease (Figs. 12 and 13), and identifying risk for glaucoma, among others.

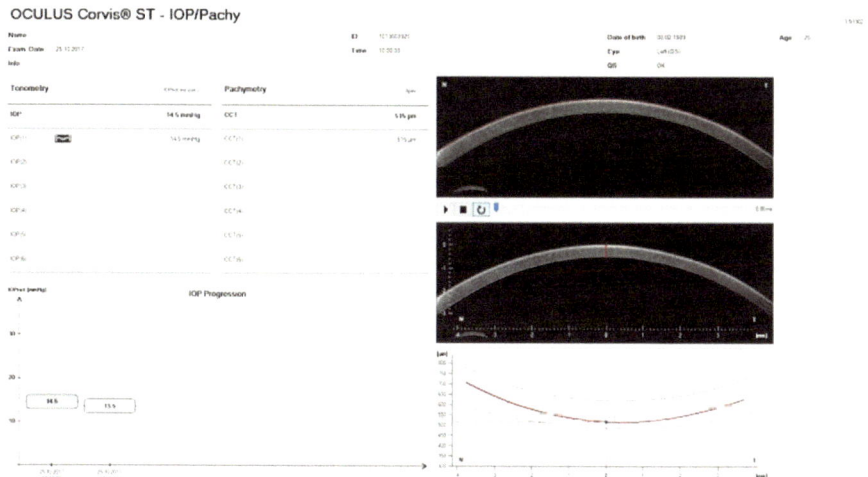

Fig. 10 Corvis ST IOP/Pachy display. On the left side of the display, we can note IOP and corneal apex pachymetry measurements and follow IOP progression comparing to previous measurements. On the right side of the display, we can observe Scheimpflug images and watch corneal displacement video

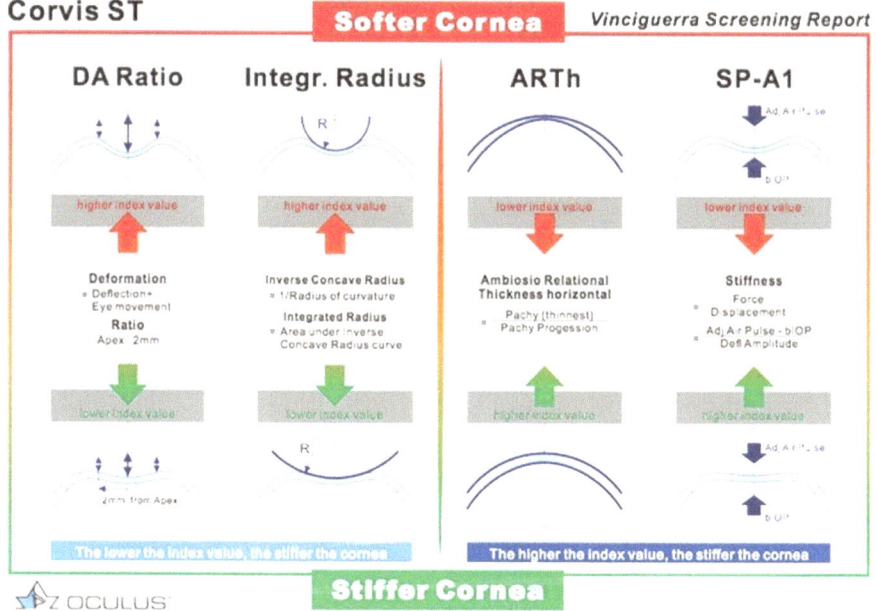

Fig. 11 Vinciguerra Screening Report: softer corneas present higher values of DA ratio and inverse concave radius while presenting lower values for ART h (Ambrósio relational thickness horizontal) and SP- A1 (stiffness parameter)

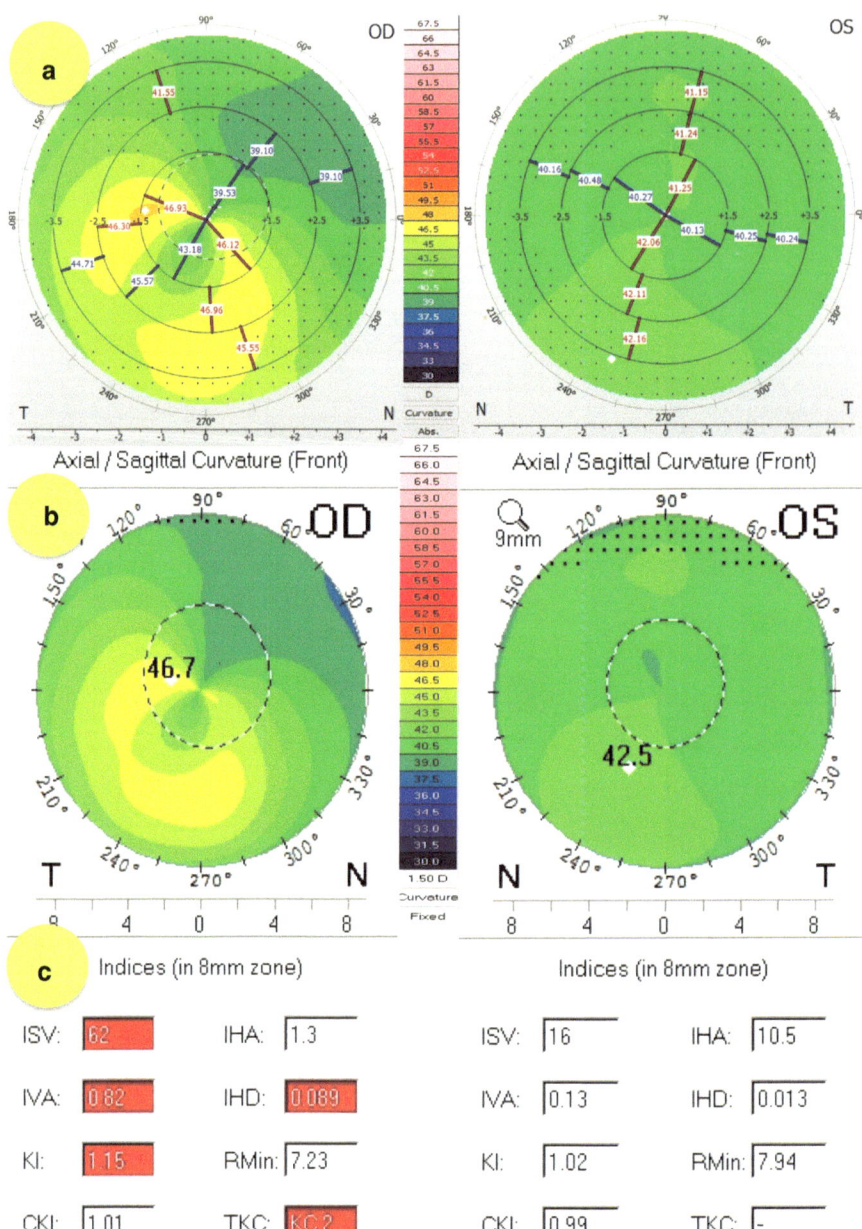

Fig. 12 Very asymmetric KC case: axial curvature maps of the front corneal surface obtained with the (**a**) Keratograph 5 M (Oculus Optikgeräte GmbH, Wetzlar, Germany), (**b**) Pentacam HR corneal tomography (Oculus Optikgeräte GmbH, Wetzlar, Germany), and (**c**) Pentacam topometric indices from both eyes. Note the classic "crab-claw" pattern in the right eye. The left eye had a relatively normal pattern with a very mild asymmetry

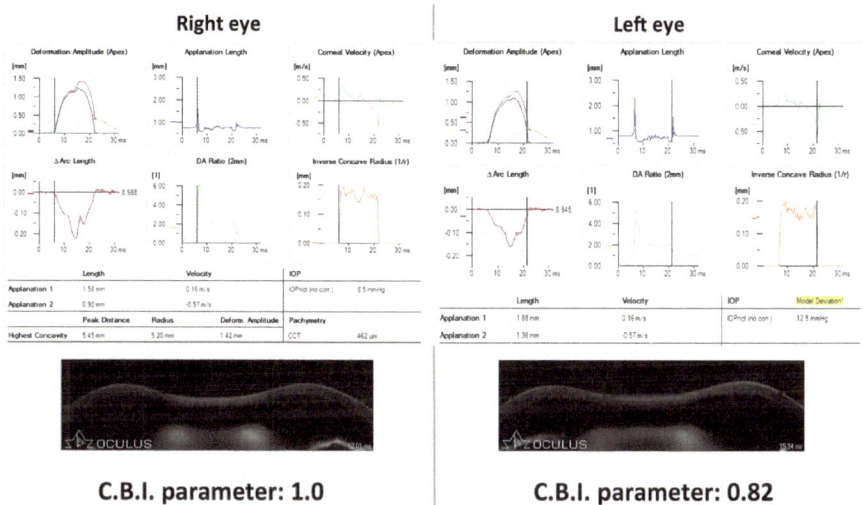

Fig. 13 Corneal deformation analysis provided by the Corvis ST. Note the abnormal CBI values of 1.00 in the right eye and 0.82 in the left eye, despite the relatively normal topographic pattern

The relevance of the application of dynamic Scheimpflug imaging for several clinical conditions was reviewed in a film produced by Ramos and coworkers (Scheimpflug Revelations, available at https://www.youtube.com/watch?v=VQj1 pVexW8c). Other authors have described other clinical applications for dynamic Scheimpflug imaging in daily practice [37, 38]. Faria-Correia and coworkers reported a case that was misdiagnosed as diffuse lamellar keratitis after LASIK, in which ocular hypertension in pressure-induced stromal keratopathy was associated with lower deformation response [38].

The ability of Corvis ST to detect ectasia has been investigated since the prototype device was tested [16], but the fact is that the first set of parameters performed relatively poorly in discriminating between normal and KC [39, 40]. An earlier study performed with the Corvis prototype retrospectively investigated the differences between normal eyes (N group); eyes with topographic patterns suspicious of KC, but with normal tomography and are stable for over 1 year (KCS group); KC eyes (KC group); and eyes with normal topographic patterns from cases with very asymmetric KC (FFKC group). Although normal individuals and those with KC showed significantly different distributions for the parameters studied, a substantial overlap was found, and the best parameter was the radius of curvature at the highest concavity (area under the curve, 0.852). Aiming to enhance the separation between the groups, the BrAIN group (Brazilian Study Group of Artificial Intelligence and Corneal Analysis) used artificial intelligence to calculate a logistic regression analysis (LRA) model with a specific combination of parameters developing the Corvis Prototype-Factor (CPF-1), which showed an AUC of 0.945. Interestingly, further statistical analysis found no differences in CPF-1 for the FFKC and KC groups and the N and KCS groups, but there were significant differences for N vs. FFKC, N vs. KC, KCS vs. FFKC, and KCS vs. KC [41].

In recent years, several other studies investigating the application of the Corvis ST for KC diagnosis have been published [39, 40, 42–48]. Interestingly, a comparative study involving normal and KC eyes found that most of the biomechanical variables from the Corvis ST, including deformation amplitude, maximum corneal inward velocity, maximum corneal outward velocity, and maximum deformation area, are significantly different between the groups [49].

In 2014, a multicenter international task force group was created with the purpose of enhancing our knowledge about Corvis ST parameters with special focus on improving their accuracy in diagnosing ectatic corneal diseases. Vinciguerra et al. used LRA to combine deformation response parameters with corneal thickness profile and developed the corneal biomechanical index (CBI) [50]. The first study included 658 patients from 2 different countries, used to create and validate the CBI parameter using 2 databases. In the training database, using a cutoff of 0.5, this index showed an AUC of 0.983, with 100% specificity and 94.1% sensitivity. Later, in the validation study, the same cutoff correctly classified 98.8% of cases, with 98.4% specificity and 100% sensitivity (Figs. 12 and 13) [50].

Integrated Parameters

Luz and coworkers evaluated the performance of the ORA and Pentacam HR (Oculus Optikgeräte GmbH, Wetzlar, Germany) integration in differentiating forme fruste keratoconus (FFKC) from normal corneas. Seventy-six eyes of 76 normal individuals and 21 eyes of 21 patients with FFKC were included in the study, which found a combination of the waveform and tomographic parameters to have the best accuracy, outperforming all individual parameters [14]. However, no integrated software was ever developed for facilitating such a clinical approach.

Interestingly, in a multicenter study, Ambrósio and coworkers introduced a new index that combined tomographic and biomechanical data for enhancing ectasia detection. The tomographic biomechanical index (TBI) was developed with artificial intelligence using the random forest method with leave-one-out cross-validation (RF/LOOCV) as the best model [13]. The study involved normal eyes (group 1; $n = 480$), KC eyes (group 2; $n = 204$), and unoperated ectatic eyes from patients with very asymmetric ectasia (group 3 very asymmetric ectasia - eye with abnormal topography (VAE-E); $n = 72$) whose fellow eyes (group 4 very asymmetric ectasia - eye with normal topography (VAE-NT); $n = 94$) showed normal topography. Using a cutoff of 0.79, TBI provided 100% sensitivity and specificity to detect clinical ectasia. In group 4, an optimized cutoff of 0.29 provided 90.4% sensitivity and 96% specificity, with an area under the ROC curve of 0.985 [13]. This study demonstrated that the TBI is more sensitive than previous parameters for detecting subclinical ectasia among eyes with normal topography in very asymmetric patients. This work was the basis for the Corvis ST and Pentacam combination in commercially available software.

External validation studies were conducted including 1 eye from 100 patients with mild keratoconus from India [48] and 24 patients with very asymmetric ectasia from Iran [51], along with a normal control group with 1 eye from 100 normal cases from India and 34 normal patients from Iran. Considering ectatic eyes, TBI showed 99% sensitivity and 100% specificity in the Indian population and 100% sensitivity and specificity in the cases from Iran. Concerning eyes with normal topography from the 24 very asymmetric ectasia cases from Iran, TBI provided 91.6% sensitivity with 97% specificity with a cutoff of 0.27 [51]. Further external validation studies also demonstrated the ability of TBI to detect keratoconus and also to distinguish mild forms of ectasia on the eyes with normal topography from patients presenting with ectasia in the fellow eye (Figs. 14, 15, and 16) [52] and also in other anecdotal cases with high susceptibility to develop ectasia, such as an identical twin sister with normal topography in both eyes of a patient with asymmetric keratoconus [53] (Figs. 17 and 18) and on the unoperated stable eye from a patient that developed unexplained ectasia after LASIK [17, 53].

Current and future studies aim to develop and expand the application of such integration method in our clinical practice, not only to augment the overall accuracy to diagnosis ectasia but to enhance treatment planning for such patients.

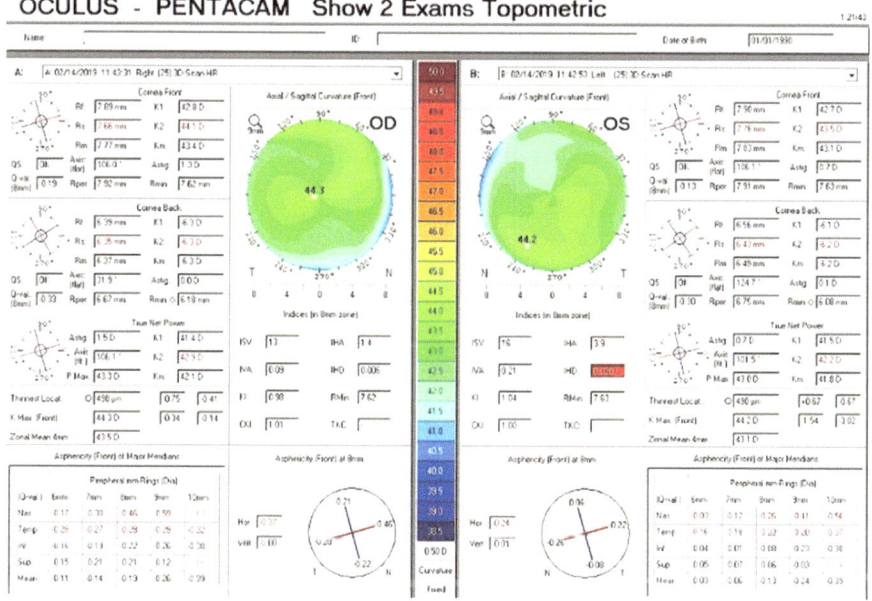

Fig. 14 Curvature maps of the front corneal surface obtained with the Pentacam HR corneal tomography (Oculus Optikgeräte GmbH, Wetzlar, Germany). Note a mild asymmetry between OD and OS

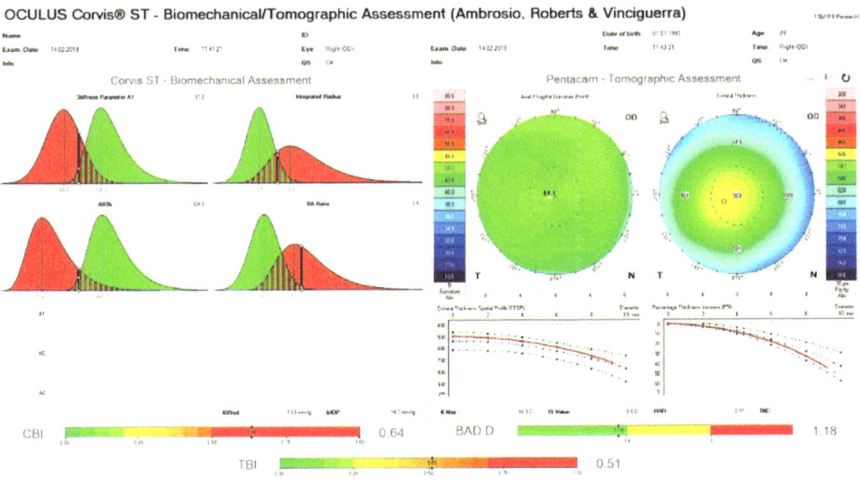

Fig. 15 TBI display from OD. Despite the relatively normal anterior curvature map, an abnormal TBI value of 0.51 was found

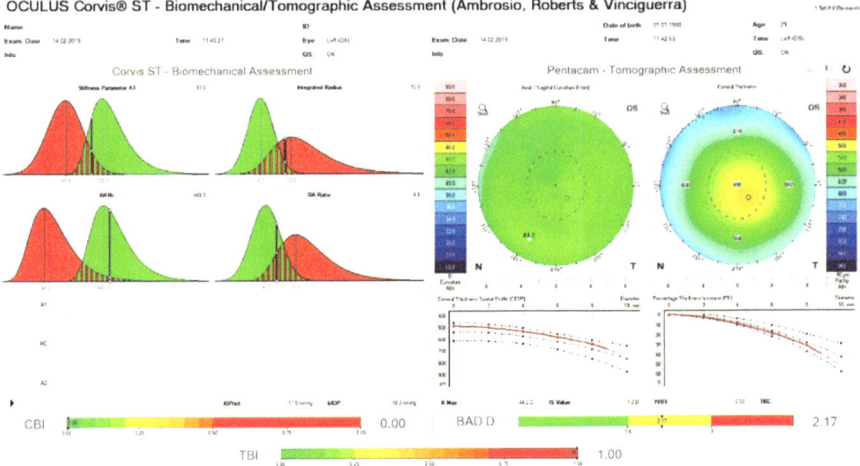

Fig. 16 TBI display from OS. An abnormal TBI value of 1.00 was found

Conclusions

The correct characterization of in vivo corneal biomechanics is still challenging because of the influence of IOP. Nevertheless, understanding corneal behavior is useful in several clinical situations including glaucoma and corneal disorders and especially in the detection of ectatic diseases [54, 55]. The integration of

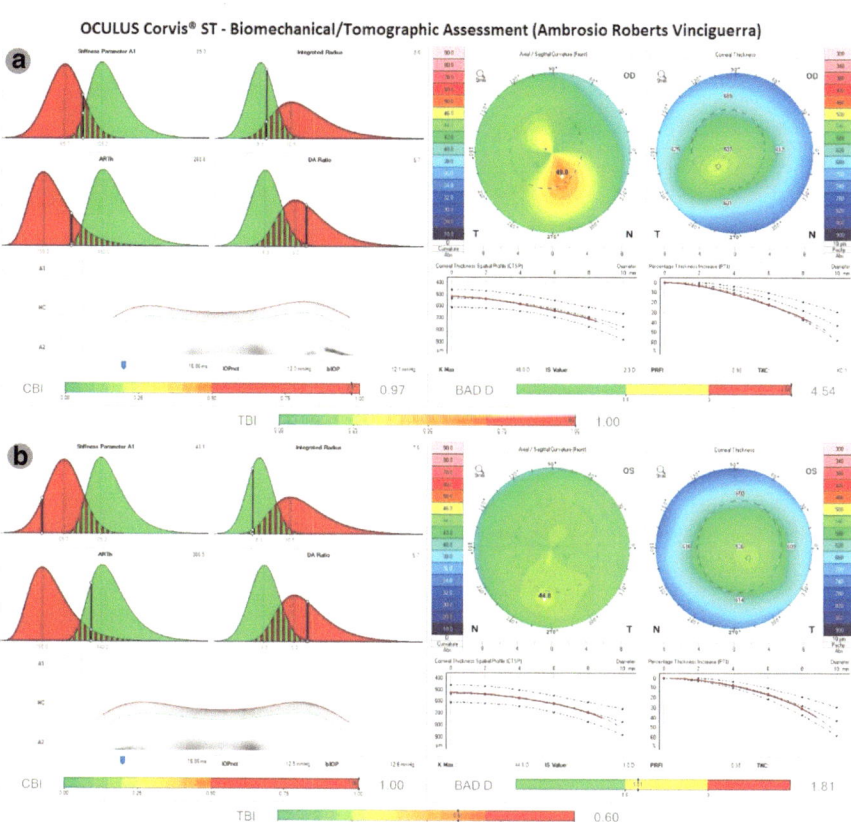

Fig. 17 (**a**) Twin 1: tomographic biomechanical display (TBI) from Pentacam and Corvis ST reveals moderate inferior steepening in OD with abnormal CBI, BAD D, and TBI values of 0.97, 4.54, and 1.00, respectively. (**b**) Twin 1: TBI display from OS demonstrates relatively normal topography but abnormal CBI, BAD D, and TBI values of 1.00, 1.81, and 0.60, respectively

biomechanical analysis with tomographic data is a reality with further promising advances. We demonstrated improvement in the accuracy to detect mild forms of KC but to also to identify an inherent predisposition to iatrogenic ectasia after laser vision correction [53]. Video 1 demonstrates a short video that mentions the main topics discussed in this chapter.

While significant improvements have been made, there is still a tremendous need for further research. Other technologies such as the noninvasive Brillouin spectroscopy are promising to add clinical information by mapping the biomechanical state of the cornea perpendicular to the surface [56, 57]. We expect continuous and further accelerated improvements in knowledge in this field.

Financial Disclosure(s) **Dr. Ambrósio is a consultant for OCULUS Optikgeräte GmbH.**

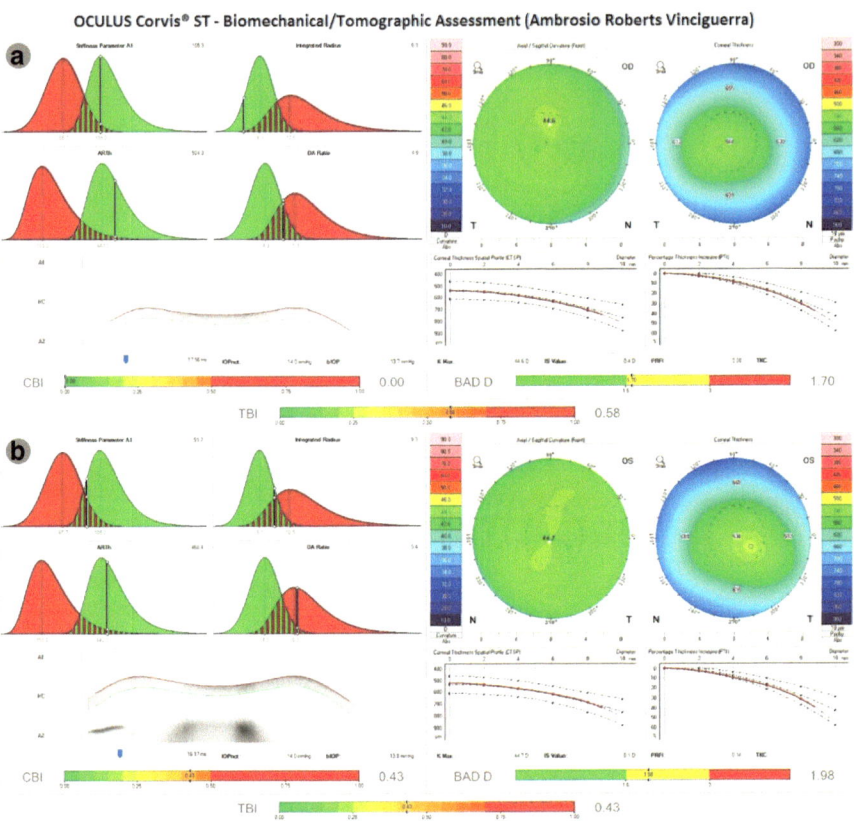

Fig. 18 (**a, b**) Twin 2: TBI displays from OD and OS demonstrating relatively normal topography in OU but abnormal BAD D (1.70 in OD and 1.98 in OS) and TBI (0.58 in OD and 0.43 in OS) values

References

1. Seiler T, Quurke AW. Iatrogenic keratectasia after LASIK in a case of forme fruste keratoconus. J Cataract Refract Surg. 1998;24:1007–9.
2. Ambrosio R Jr, Randleman JB. Screening for ectasia risk: what are we screening for and how should we screen for it? J Refract Surg (Thorofare, NJ : 1995). 2013;29:230–2.
3. Binder PS. Ectasia after laser in situ keratomileusis. J Cataract Refract Surg. 2003;29:2419–29.
4. McGhee CN, Kim BZ, Wilson PJ. Contemporary treatment paradigms in keratoconus. Cornea. 2015;34(Suppl 10):S16–23.
5. Ambrosio R Jr, Faria-Correia F, Silva-Lopes I, Azevedo- Wagner A, Tanos FW, Lopes B, Salomão M. Paradigms, paradoxes and controversies on keratoconus and corneal ectatic diseases. Int J Keratoconus Ectatic Corneal Dis. 2018;7:35–49.
6. Maeda N, Klyce SD, Smolek MK, Thompson HW. Automated keratoconus screening with corneal topography analysis. Invest Ophthalmol Vis Sci. 1994;35:2749–57.
7. Maguire LJ, Bourne WM. Corneal topography of early keratoconus. Am J Ophthalmol. 1989;108:107–12.

8. Ambrosio R Jr, Valbon BF, Faria-Correia F, Ramos I, Luz A. Scheimpflug imaging for laser refractive surgery. Curr Opin Ophthalmol. 2013;24:310–20.

9. Smadja D, Touboul D, Cohen A, Doveh E, Santhiago MR, Mello GR, et al. Detection of subclinical keratoconus using an automated decision tree classification. Am J Ophthalmol. 2013;156:237–46.e1.

10. Saad A, Gatinel D. Topographic and tomographic properties of forme fruste keratoconus corneas. Invest Ophthalmol Vis Sci. 2010;51:5546–55.

11. Golan O, Piccinini AL, Hwang ES, De Oca Gonzalez IM, Krauthammer M, Khandelwal SS, et al. Distinguishing highly asymmetric keratoconus eyes using dual Scheimpflug/placido analysis. Am J Ophthalmol. 2019;201:46.

12. Hwang ES, Perez-Straziota CE, Kim SW, Santhiago MR, Randleman JB. Distinguishing highly asymmetric keratoconus eyes using combined Scheimpflug and spectral-domain OCT analysis. Ophthalmology. 2018;125:1862–71.

13. Ambrosio R Jr, Lopes BT, Faria-Correia F, Salomao MQ, Buhren J, Roberts CJ, et al. Integration of Scheimpflug-based corneal tomography and biomechanical assessments for enhancing ectasia detection. J Refract Surg (Thorofare, NJ : 1995). 2017;33.434–43.

14. Luz A, Lopes B, Hallahan KM, Valbon B, Ramos I, Faria-Correia F, et al. Enhanced combined tomography and biomechanics data for distinguishing forme fruste keratoconus. J Refract Surg (Thorofare, NJ : 1995). 2016;32:479–94.

15. Ambrosio R Jr, Belin M. Enhanced screening for ectasia risk prior to laser vision correction. Int J Keratoconus Ectatic Corneal Dis. 2017;6:23–33.

16. Ambrosio R Jr, Nogueira LP, Caldas DL, Fontes BM, Luz A, Cazal JO, et al. Evaluation of corneal shape and biomechanics before LASIK. Int Ophthalmol Clin. 2011;51:11–38.

17. Ambrósio Junior R, Caldas DL, RSD S, Pimentel LN, BDF V. Impacto da análise do "wavefront" na refratometria de pacientes com ceratocone. Rev Bras Oftalmol. 2010;69:294–300.

18. Gomes JA, Tan D, Rapuano CJ, Belin MW, Ambrosio R Jr, Guell JL, et al. Global consensus on keratoconus and ectatic diseases. Cornea. 2015;34:359–69.

19. Roberts CJ, Dupps WJ Jr. Biomechanics of corneal ectasia and biomechanical treatments. J Cataract Refract Surg. 2014;40:991–8.

20. Salomão M, Hoffling-Lima AL, Lopes B, Belin MW, Sena N, Dawson DG, et al. Recent developments in keratoconus diagnosis. Exp Rev Ophthalmol. 2018;13:329–41.

21. Luce DA. Determining in vivo biomechanical properties of the cornea with an ocular response analyzer. J Cataract Refract Surg. 2005;31:156–62.

22. Roberts CJ. Concepts and misconceptions in corneal biomechanics. J Cataract Refract Surg. 2014;40:862–9.

23. Pinero DP, Alcon N. In vivo characterization of corneal biomechanics. J Cataract Refract Surg. 2014;40:870–87.

24. Shah S, Laiquzzaman M, Bhojwani R, Mantry S, Cunliffe I. Assessment of the biomechanical properties of the cornea with the ocular response analyzer in normal and keratoconic eyes. Invest Ophthalmol Vis Sci. 2007;48:3026–31.

25. Shah S, Laiquzzaman M. Comparison of corneal biomechanics in pre and post-refractive surgery and keratoconic eyes by ocular response analyser. Contact Lens Anterior Eye: J Br Contact Lens Assoc. 2009;32:129–32. quiz 51

26. Fontes BM, Ambrosio Junior R, Jardim D, Velarde GC, Nose W. Ability of corneal biomechanical metrics and anterior segment data in the differentiation of keratoconus and healthy corneas. Arq Bras Oftalmol. 2010;73:333–7.

27. Fontes BM, Ambrosio R Jr, Jardim D, Velarde GC, Nose W. Corneal biomechanical metrics and anterior segment parameters in mild keratoconus. Ophthalmology. 2010;117:673–9.

28. Galletti JD, Ruisenor Vazquez PR, Fuentes Bonthoux F, Pfortner T, Galletti JG. Multivariate analysis of the ocular response analyzer's corneal deformation response curve for early keratoconus detection. J Ophthalmol. 2015;2015:496382.

29. Hallahan KM, Sinha Roy A, Ambrosio R Jr, Salomao M, Dupps WJ Jr. Discriminant value of custom ocular response analyzer waveform derivatives in keratoconus. Ophthalmology. 2014;121:459–68.

30. Ventura BV, Machado AP, Ambrosio R Jr, Ribeiro G, Araujo LN, Luz A, et al. Analysis of waveform-derived ORA parameters in early forms of keratoconus and normal corneas. J Refract Surg (Thorofare, NJ : 1995). 2013;29:637–43.

31. Luz A, Fontes BM, Lopes B, Ramos I, Schor P, Ambrosio R Jr. ORA waveform-derived biomechanical parameters to distinguish normal from keratoconic eyes. Arq Bras Oftalmol. 2013;76:111–7.

32. Mikielewicz M, Kotliar K, Barraquer RI, Michael R. Air-pulse corneal applanation signal curve parameters for the characterisation of keratoconus. Br J Ophthalmol. 2011;95:793–8.

33. Ambrosio R Jr, Ramos I, Luz A, Faria-Correia F, Steinmueller A, Krug M, et al. Dynamic ultra-high speed Scheimpflug imaging for assessing corneal biomechanical properties. Rev Bras Oftalmol. 2013;72:99.

34. Bao F, Deng M, Wang Q, Huang J, Yang J, Whitford C, et al. Evaluation of the relationship of corneal biomechanical metrics with physical intraocular pressure and central corneal thickness in ex vivo rabbit eye globes. Exp Eye Res. 2015;137:11–7.

35. Bao F, Huang Z, Huang J, Wang J, Deng M, Li L, et al. Clinical evaluation of methods to correct intraocular pressure measurements by the Goldmann applanation tonometer, ocular response analyzer, and Corvis ST tonometer for the effects of corneal stiffness parameters. J Glaucoma. 2016;25:510–9.

36. Joda AA, Shervin MM, Kook D, Elsheikh A. Development and validation of a correction equation for Corvis tonometry. Comput Methods Biomech Biomed Engin. 2016;19:943–53.

37. Valbon BF, Ambrosio R Jr, Fontes BM, Alves MR. Effects of age on corneal deformation by non-contact tonometry integrated with an ultra-high-speed (UHS) Scheimpflug camera. Arq Bras Oftalmol. 2013;76:229–32.

38. Faria-Correia F, Ramos I, Valbon B, Luz A, Roberts CJ, Ambrosio R Jr. Scheimpflug-based tomography and biomechanical assessment in pressure-induced stromal keratopathy. J Refract Surg. 2013;29:356–8.

39. Ali NQ, Patel DV, McGhee CN. Biomechanical responses of healthy and keratoconic corneas measured using a noncontact scheimpflug-based tonometer. Invest Ophthalmol Vis Sci. 2014;55:3651–9.

40. Steinberg J, Katz T, Lucke K, Frings A, Druchkiv V, Linke SJ. Screening for keratoconus with new dynamic biomechanical in vivo Scheimpflug analyses. Cornea. 2015;34:1404–12.

41. Salomão MQ, Faria-Correa F, Ramos I, Luz A, Ambrósio RJ. Corneal deformation response with dynamic ultra-high-speed scheimpflug imaging for detecting ectatic corneas. Int J Keratoconus Ectatic Corneal Dis. 2016;5:1–5.

42. Bak-Nielsen S, Pedersen IB, Ivarsen A, Hjortdal J. Dynamic Scheimpflug-based assessment of keratoconus and the effects of corneal cross-linking. J Refract Surg. 2014;30:408–14.

43. Tian L, Huang YF, Wang LQ, Bai H, Wang Q, Jiang JJ, et al. Corneal biomechanical assessment using corneal visualization scheimpflug technology in keratoconic and normal eyes. J Ophthalmol. 2014;2014:147516.

44. Koprowski R, Ambrosio R Jr. Quantitative assessment of corneal vibrations during intraocular pressure measurement with the air-puff method in patients with keratoconus. Comput Biol Med. 2015;66:170–8.

45. Pena-Garcia P, Peris-Martinez C, Abbouda A, Ruiz-Moreno JM. Detection of subclinical keratoconus through non-contact tonometry and the use of discriminant biomechanical functions. J Biomech. 2016;49:353–63.

46. Wang LK, Tian L, Zheng YP. Determining in vivo elasticity and viscosity with dynamic Scheimpflug imaging analysis in keratoconic and healthy eyes. J Biophotonics. 2016;9:454.

47. Sedaghat MR, Momeni-Moghaddam H, Ambrosio R Jr, Heidari HR, Maddah N, Danesh Z, et al. Diagnostic ability of corneal shape and biomechanical parameters for detecting frank keratoconus. Cornea. 2018;37:1025–34.

48. Kataria P, Padmanabhan P, Gopalakrishnan A, Padmanaban V, Mahadik S, Ambrosio R Jr. Accuracy of Scheimpflug-derived corneal biomechanical and tomographic indices for detecting subclinical and mild keratectasia in a south Asian population. J Cataract Refract Surg. 2018;45:328.
49. Tian L, Ko MW, Wang LK, Zhang JY, Li TJ, Huang YF, et al. Assessment of ocular biomechanics using dynamic ultra high-speed Scheimpflug imaging in keratoconic and normal eyes. J Refract Surg. 2014;30:785–91.
50. Vinciguerra R, Ambrosio R Jr, Elsheikh A, Roberts CJ, Lopes B, Morenghi E, et al. Detection of keratoconus with a new biomechanical index. J Refract Surg (Thorofare, NJ : 1995). 2016;32:803–10.
51. Sedaghat MR, Momeni-Moghaddam H, Ambrosio R Jr, Roberts CJ, Yekta AA, Danesh Z, et al. Long-term evaluation of corneal biomechanical properties after corneal cross-linking for keratoconus: a 4-year longitudinal study. J Refract Surg (Thorofare, NJ : 1995). 2018;34:849–56.
52. Ferreira-Mendes J, Lopes BT, Faria-Correia F, Salomao MQ, Rodrigues-Barros S, Ambrosio R Jr. Enhanced ectasia detection using corneal tomography and biomechanics. Am J Ophthalmol. 2019;197:7–16.
53. Salomao MQ, Hofling-Lima AL, Faria-Correia F, Lopes BT, Rodrigues-Barros S, Roberts CJ, et al. Dynamic corneal deformation response and integrated corneal tomography. Indian J Ophthalmol. 2018;66:373–82.
54. Dupps WJ Jr, Roberts CJ. Corneal biomechanics: a decade later. J Cataract Refract Surg. 2014;40:857.
55. Dupps WJ Jr, Wilson SE. Biomechanics and wound healing in the cornea. Exp Eye Res. 2006;83:709–20.
56. Seiler TG, Shao P, Eltony A, Seiler T, Yun SH. Brillouin spectroscopy of normal and keratoconus corneas. Am J Ophthalmol. 2019;202:118.
57. Yun SH, Chernyak D. Brillouin microscopy: assessing ocular tissue biomechanics. Curr Opin Ophthalmol. 2018;29:299–305.

Corneal Topography, Corneal Tomography, and Epithelial Maps in Keratoconus

Dan Z. Reinstein, Timothy J. Archer, Ryan S. Vida, Ronald H. Silverman, and Raksha Urs

Introduction

Keratoconus (KC) is a progressive, corneal dystrophy which manifests as corneal thinning and formation of a cone-shaped protrusion. Because laser refractive surgery may lead to accelerated postoperative ectasia in patients with keratoconus [1, 2], the accurate detection of early keratoconus is a major safety concern. The prevalence of keratoconus in the Caucasian population is approximately 1/2000 [3]. The incidence of undiagnosed keratoconus presenting to refractive surgery clinics tends to be much higher than this, as keratoconics develop astigmatism that is more difficult to correct by contact lenses or glasses, leading them to consider refractive surgery [4]. The challenge for keratoconus screening is to have high sensitivity, but this has to be combined with high specificity to minimize the number of atypical normal patients who are denied surgery.

Electronic Supplementary Material The online version of this chapter (https://doi. org/10.1007/978-3-030-66143-4_3) contains supplementary material, which is available to authorized users.

D. Z. Reinstein (✉)
London Vision Clinic, London, UK

Columbia University Medical Center, New York, NY, USA

Sorbonne Université, Paris, France

School of Biomedical Sciences, University of Ulster, Coleraine, UK
e-mail: dzr@londonvisionclinic.com

T. J. Archer · R. S. Vida
London Vision Clinic, London, UK

R. H. Silverman · R. Urs
Columbia University Medical Center, New York, NY, USA

© Springer Nature Switzerland AG 2021
C. Carriazo, M. J. Cosentino (eds.), *New Frontiers for the Treatment of Keratoconus*, https://doi.org/10.1007/978-3-030-66143-4_3

27

There have been significant efforts made to develop methods for screening of early keratoconus over the last 30 years. In 1984, Klyce [5] introduced color-coded maps derived from computerized front surface Placido topography, which have made the diagnosis of keratoconus easier, as patterns including inferior steepening, asymmetric bow-tie, and skew bow-tie typical of keratoconus can be seen early in the progression of the disease [6, 7]. Placido-based instruments producing maps of anterior surface topography and curvature became available by the early 1990s, and their use in keratoconus screening has been demonstrated [7–16]. Characterization of corneal thickness and topography of both corneal surfaces using scanning-slit tomography was introduced commercially in the mid-1990s by the Orbscan scanning-slit system (Bausch & Lomb, Rochester, NY) [17–19] and later by the Pentacam rotating Scheimpflug-based system (Oculus Optikgeräte, Wetzlar, Germany) [20, 21] and other tomography scanners. Wavefront assessment [22] and the ocular response analyzer (Reichert, Depew, NY) [23] have been employed as a means for detecting early keratoconus.

Topographic and tomographic evaluation has evolved from qualitative observation [7] to quantitative measurements, and many parameters have been described to aid the differentiation of normal from keratoconic eyes [7–16]. Several statistical and machine-based or computerized learning models have been employed for keratoconus detection, and automated systems for screening based on front and back surface topography and whole corneal tomography and pachymetric profile have been developed [20, 24–31].

Although these approaches have improved the effectiveness of keratoconus screening, there are still equivocal cases where a confident diagnosis cannot be made and undiagnosed keratoconus probably remains the leading cause of corneal ectasia after LASIK [32–44]. The addition of quantitative parameters that are independent of those now obtained by topographic and tomographic analysis could potentially improve screening.

The corneal epithelial and stromal thickness profiles may represent such an independent parameter and will be the focus of this chapter. As will be described below, the corneal epithelium has the ability to alter its thickness profile to re-establish a smooth, symmetrical optical outer corneal surface and either partially or totally mask the presence of an irregular stromal surface from front surface topography [45, 46]. Therefore, the epithelial thickness profile would be expected to follow a distinctive pattern in keratoconus to partially compensate for the cone.

Epithelial Thickness Profile in Normal Eyes

All of the epithelial thickness data that is described in this chapter was obtained using the Artemis Insight 100 very high-frequency digital ultrasound arc-scanner (ArcScan Inc., Golden, CO), which has been previously described in detail [47–49].

We set out to characterize the in vivo epithelial thickness profile in a population of normal eyes with no ocular pathology other than refractive error. We obtained the epithelial thickness profile across the central 10 mm diameter of the cornea for 110 normal eyes of 56 patients and averaged the data in the population. Epithelial thickness values for left eyes were reflected in the vertical axis and superimposed onto the right eye values so that nasal/temporal characteristics could be combined [49].

The average epithelial thickness map revealed that the epithelium was not a homogeneous layer as had previously been thought but followed a very distinct pattern (Fig. 1); on average, the epithelium was 5.7 μm thicker inferiorly than superiorly and 1.2 μm thicker temporally than nasally. The pattern of thicker epithelium inferiorly than superiorly and thicker epithelium nasally than temporally was consistent across a majority of eyes in the population sampled. The average central epithelial thickness was 53.4 μm, and the standard deviation was only 4.6 μm [49]. This indicated that there was little variation in central epithelial thickness in the population. The thinnest epithelial point within the central 5 mm of the cornea was displaced on average 0.33 mm (±1.08) temporally and 0.90 mm (±0.96) superiorly with reference to the corneal vertex (Fig. 2). The epithelium appears regular, in a B-scan of a normal cornea (Fig. 3).

Figure 4, Column 1 shows the keratometry, Atlas 995 (Carl Zeiss Meditec, Jena, Germany) corneal topography map and PathFinder™ corneal analysis, Orbscan II (software version 3.00) anterior elevation Best Fit Sphere (BFS), Orbscan II posterior elevation BFS, and Artemis epithelial thickness profile of a normal eye.

Epithelial thickness can now also be measured using optical coherence tomography (OCT) systems, notably the RTVue/Avanti (OptoVue, Fremont, CA) and MS-39

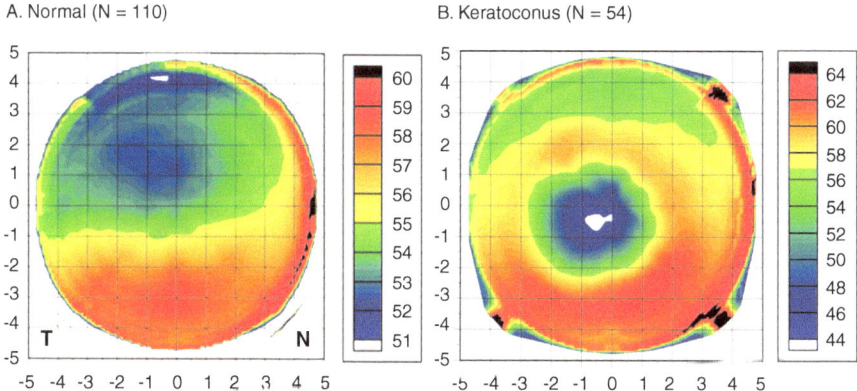

Fig. 1 Mean epithelial thickness profile for a population of 110 normal eyes (**a**) and a population of 54 keratoconic eyes (**b**). The epithelial thickness profiles for all eyes in each population were averaged using mirrored left eye symmetry. The color scale represents epithelial thickness in microns. A Cartesian 1 mm grid is superimposed with the origin at the corneal vertex. (Reprinted with permission from SLACK Incorporated: Reinstein et al. [60])

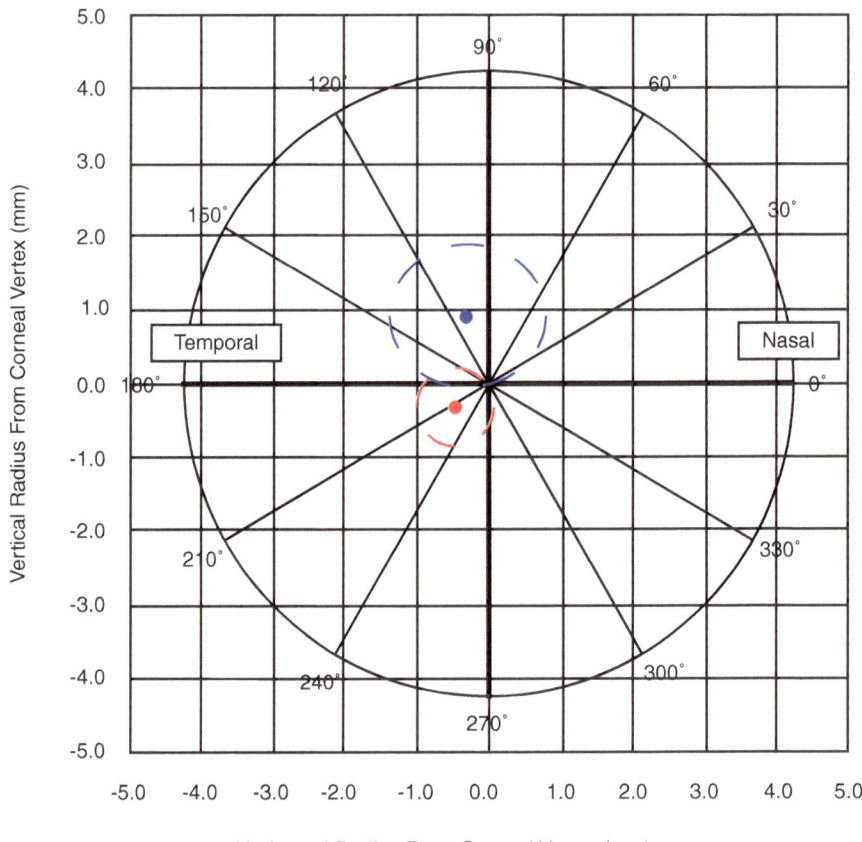

Fig. 2 Plot showing the mean location of the thinnest epithelium in a population of 110 normal eyes and 54 keratoconic eyes. The blue dot represents the mean location of the thinnest point for the normal population, and the dotted blue line represents one standard deviation. The red dot represents the mean location of the thinnest point for the keratoconic population, and the dotted red line represents one standard deviation. (Reprinted with permission from SLACK Incorporated: Reinstein et al. [60])

(CSO, Florence, Italy) [50–52]. These studies have confirmed this superior-inferior and nasal-temporal asymmetric profile for epithelial thickness in normal eyes [52].

This normal non-uniformity seems to provide evidence that the epithelial thickness is regulated by eyelid mechanics and blinking, as we suggested in 1994 [53]. The eyelid might effectively be chafing the surface epithelium during blinking and that the posterior surface of the semi-rigid tarsus provides a template for the outer shape of the epithelial surface. During blinking, which occurs on average between 300 and 1500 times per hour [54], the vertical traverse of the upper lid is much greater than that of the lower lid. Doane [55] studied the dynamics of eyelid anatomy during blinking and found that during a blink, the descent of the upper eyelid reaches its maximum speed at about the time it crosses the visual axis. As a

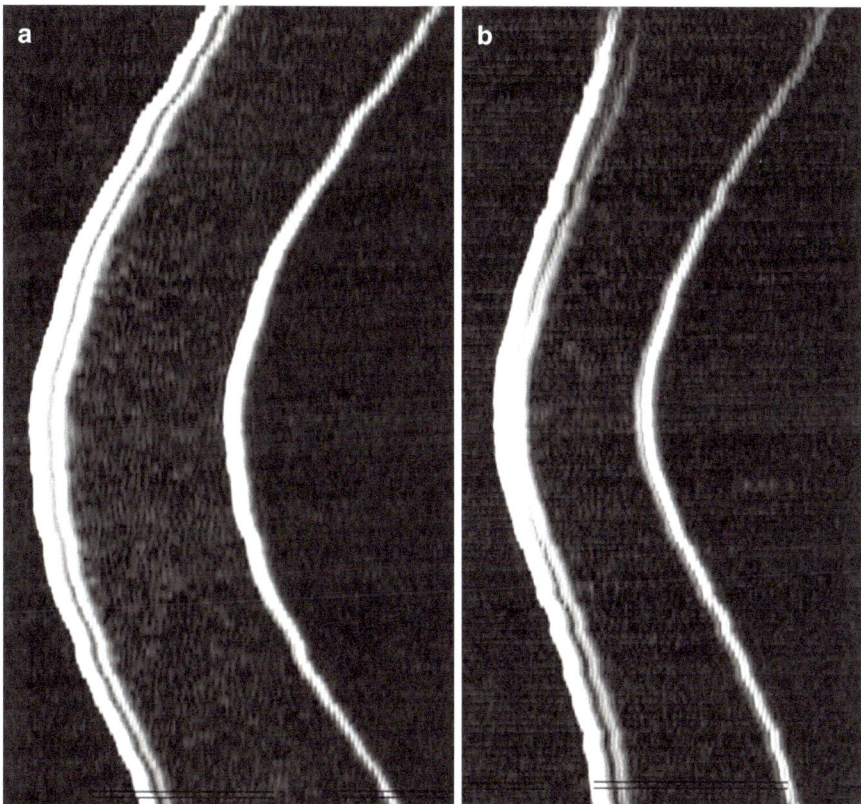

Fig. 3 (**a**) Horizontal non-geometrically corrected B-scan of a normal cornea obtained using the Artemis very high-frequency digital ultrasound arc-scanner. The epithelium appears uniform in thickness across the 10 mm diameter of the scan. (**b**) Vertical non-geometrically corrected B-scan of a keratoconic cornea obtained using the Artemis very high-frequency digital ultrasound arc-scanner. The epithelium appears very thin centrally coincident with a visible cone on the back surface. The epithelium is clearly thicker either side of the cone. The central epithelium is much thinner, and the peripheral epithelium is much thicker compared to that seen in the normal eye

consequence, it is likely that the eyelid applies more force on the superior cornea than the inferior cornea. Similarly, the friction on the cornea during lid closure is likely to be greater temporally than nasally as the outer canthus is higher than the inner canthus (mean intercanthal angle = 3°), and the temporal portion of the lid is higher than the nasal lid (mean upper lid angle = 2.7°) [56]. Therefore, it seems that the nature of the eyelid completely explains the non-uniform epithelial thickness profile of a normal eye.

Further evidence for this theory is provided by the epithelial thickness changes observed in orthokeratology [57]. In orthokeratology, a shaped contact lens is placed on the cornea overnight that sits tightly on the cornea centrally but leaves a gap in the mid-periphery. Therefore, the natural template provided by the posterior surface

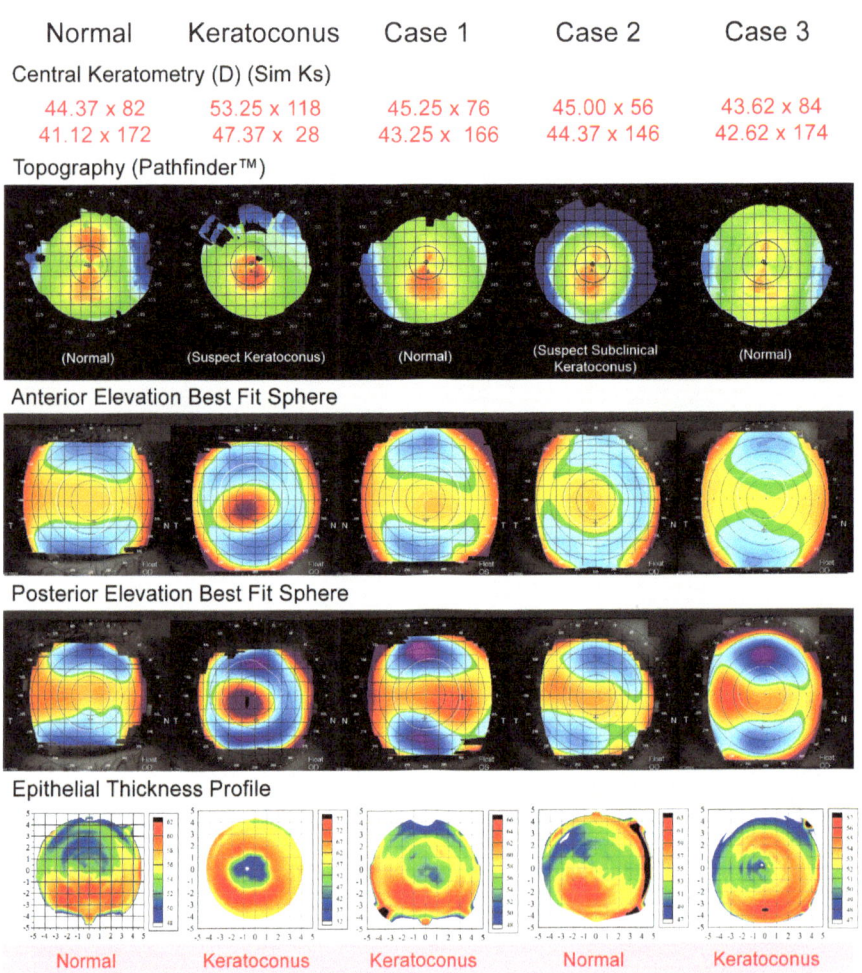

Fig. 4 Central keratometry, Atlas corneal topography and PathFinder™ corneal analysis, Orbscan anterior and posterior elevation BFS, and Artemis epithelial thickness profile for one normal eye, one keratoconic eye, and three example eyes where the diagnosis of keratoconus might be misleading from topography. The final diagnosis based on the epithelial thickness profile is shown at the bottom of each example. (Reprinted with permission from SLACK Incorporated: Reinstein et al. [60])

of the semi-rigid tarsus of the eyelid is replaced by an artificial contact lens template designed to fit tightly to the center of the cornea and loosely paracentrally. We found significant epithelial thickness changes with central thinning and mid-peripheral thickening showing that the epithelium had remodelled according to the template provided by the contact lens – i.e., the epithelium is chafed and squashed by the lens centrally, while the epithelium is free to thicken paracentrally where the lens is not so tightly fitted.

Epithelial Thickness Profile in Keratoconic Eyes

It is well known that the epithelial thickness changes in keratoconus since extreme steepening leads to epithelial breakdown, as often seen clinically. Epithelial thinning over the cone has been demonstrated using histopathologic analysis of keratoconic corneas by Scroggs et al. [58] and later using custom software and a Humphrey-Zeiss OCT system (Humphrey Systems, Dublin, Calif) by Haque et al. [59]

We have characterized the in vivo epithelial thickness profile in a population of keratoconic eyes. The subjects included for the study had previously been diagnosed with keratoconus, and the diagnosis was confirmed by clinical signs of keratoconus such as microscopic signs at the slit-lamp, corneal topographic changes, high refractive astigmatism, reduced best-corrected visual acuity and contrast sensitivity, and significant level of higher-order aberrations, in particular vertical coma. We measured the epithelial thickness profile across the central 10 mm diameter of the cornea for 54 keratoconic eyes of 30 patients and averaged the data in the population [60]. Epithelial thickness values for left eyes were reflected in the vertical axis and superimposed onto the right eye values so that nasal/temporal characteristics could be combined.

The average epithelial thickness profile in keratoconus revealed there was significantly more irregularity compared to a normal population. The epithelium was thinnest at the apex of the cone, and this thin epithelial zone was surrounded by an annulus of thickened epithelium (see Fig. 1). While all eyes exhibited the same epithelial doughnut pattern, characterized by a localized central zone of thinning surrounded by an annulus of thick epithelium, the thickness values of the thinnest point and the thickest point as well as the difference in thickness between the thinnest and thickest epithelium varied greatly between eyes. There was a statistically significant correlation between the thinnest epithelium and the steepest keratometry (D), indicating that as the cornea became steeper, the epithelial thickness minimum became thinner. In addition, there was a statistically significant correlation between the thickness of the thinnest epithelium and the difference in thickness between the thinnest and thickest epithelium. This indicated that as the epithelium thinned, there was an increase in the irregularity of the epithelial thickness profile – i.e., that there was an increase in the severity of the keratoconus. The location of the thinnest epithelium within the central 5 mm of the cornea was displaced on average 0.48 mm (± 0.66 mm) temporally and 0.32 mm (±0.67 mm) inferiorly with reference to the corneal vertex (Fig. 2). The mean epithelial thickness for all eyes was 45.7 ± 5.9 μm (range 33.1–56.3 μm) at the corneal vertex, 38.2 ± 5.8 μm (range 29.6–52.4 μm) at the thinnest point, and 66.8 ± 7.2 μm (range 54.1–94.4 μm) at the thickest point [60].

Figure 3 shows a B-scan for a keratoconic cornea which demonstrates the lack of homogeneity in epithelial thickness as well as central corneal thinning. There is epithelial thinning over the cone and relative epithelial thickening adjacent to the stromal surface cone.

Figure 4, Column 2 shows the keratometry, Atlas 995 corneal topography map and PathFinder™ corneal analysis, Orbscan II anterior elevation BFS, Orbscan II posterior elevation BFS, and Artemis epithelial thickness profile of a keratoconic eye. As expected, the front surface topography shows inferotemporal steepening with steep average keratometry and high astigmatism; the anterior and posterior elevation BFS maps demonstrate that the apex of the cone is located inferotemporally; the epithelial thickness profile shows epithelial thinning at the apex of the cone surrounded by an annulus of thicker epithelium. The steepest cornea coincides with the apex of the anterior and posterior elevation BFS as well as with the location of the thinnest epithelium.

The epithelial thickness profile for keratoconus as described here has been confirmed by studies using OCT [52, 61–63]. The study by Laroche's group [63] elegantly described the different stages of advanced keratoconus demonstrating that as keratoconus moves into its latter stages, a very different epithelial thickness profile becomes apparent. In advanced keratoconus, there is stromal loss often in the location of the cone, for example, due to hydrops. This means that rather than the cone being elevated relative to the rest of the stroma, this region is now a depression. Therefore, the epithelium changes from being thinnest over the cone to being thickest in this region, as it is compensating for a depression instead of an elevation (see next section). There can be significant stromal loss in such advanced keratoconus, so the epithelium can be as thick as 200 μm in some cases. Examples of this epithelial thickening were also reported by Rocha et al. [61] who concluded that focal central epithelial thinning was suggestive but not pathognomonic for keratoconus (i.e., the presence of an epithelial doughnut pattern did not prove beyond any doubt that an eye has keratoconus). However, as described by Laroche, these cases only appear in very advanced keratoconus, which means that they are of no interest with respect to keratoconus screening. Eyes with early keratoconus will never present with epithelial thickening in the location of the cone as by definition if there has been stromal loss, then the keratoconus must be more advanced and the cornea will be obviously abnormal.

Understanding the Predictable Behavior of the Corneal Epithelium

Epithelial thickness changes in keratoconus provide another example of the very predictable mechanism of the corneal epithelium to compensate for irregularities on the stromal surface. Epithelial thickness changes have also been described after myopic excimer laser ablation [64–67], hyperopic excimer laser ablation [68], radial keratotomy [69], and intracorneal ring segments [70] and in irregularly irregular astigmatism after corneal refractive surgery [45, 71–75] and in ectasia [76].

In all of these cases, the epithelial thickness changes are clearly a compensatory response to the change in the stromal surface and can all be explained by the theory of eyelid template regulation of epithelial thickness [46]. Compensatory epithelial thickness changes can be summarized by the following rules:

1. The epithelium thickens in areas where tissue has been removed or the curvature has been flattened (e.g., central thickening after myopic ablation [64–66] or radial keratotomy [69] and peripheral thickening after hyperopic ablation [68]).
2. The epithelium thins over regions that are relatively elevated or the curvature has been steepened (e.g., central thinning in keratoconus [52, 60–63] and ectasia [76] and after hyperopic ablation [68]).
3. The magnitude of epithelial changes correlates to the magnitude of the change in curvature (e.g., more epithelial thickening after higher myopic ablation [64, 65, 67], after higher hyperopic ablation [68], and in more advanced keratoconus [52, 60–63]).
4. The amount of epithelial remodelling is defined by the rate of change of curvature of an irregularity [46, 77]; there will be more epithelial remodelling for a more localized irregularity [45, 72, 73, 75]. The epithelium effectively acts as a low-pass filter, smoothing local changes (high curvature gradient) almost completely, but only partially smoothing global changes (low curvature gradient). For example, there is almost twice as much epithelial thickening after a hyperopic ablation [68] compared with a myopic ablation [64, 65, 67], and there is almost total epithelial compensation for small, very localized stromal loss such as after a corneal ulcer [68].

Diagnosing Early Keratoconus Using Epithelial Thickness Profiles

Mapping of the epithelial thickness reveals a very distinct thickness profile in keratoconus compared to that of normal corneas, due to the compensatory mechanism of the epithelium for stromal irregularities. The epithelial thickness profile changes with the progression of the disease; as the keratoconus becomes more severe, the epithelium at the apex of the cone becomes thinner, and the surrounding annulus of the epithelium in the epithelial doughnut pattern becomes thicker. Therefore, the degree of epithelial abnormality in both directions (thinner and thicker than normal) can be used to confirm or exclude a diagnosis of keratoconus in eyes suggestive but not conclusive of a diagnosis of keratoconus on topography at a very early stage in the expression of the disease [78].

Pattern of Epithelial Thickness Profile

The epithelial thickness profile in normal eyes demonstrates that the epithelium is on average thicker inferiorly than superiorly and slightly thicker nasally than temporally. There is very little variation in epithelial thickness within both the inferior hemi-cornea and the superior hemi-cornea. In contrast, in keratoconic eyes, the average epithelial thickness map showed an epithelial doughnut pattern characterized by a localized central zone of thinning overlying the stromal cone, surrounded by an annulus of thick epithelium. In early keratoconus, we would expect to see the pattern of localized epithelial thinning surrounded by an annulus of thick epithelium coincident with a suspected cone on posterior elevation BFS. The coincidence of epithelial thinning together with an eccentric posterior elevation BFS apex may reveal whether or not to ascribe significance to an eccentric posterior elevation BFS apex occurring *concurrently with* a normal front surface topography. In other words, in the presence of normal or questionable front surface topography, thinning of the epithelium coincident with the location of the posterior elevation BFS apex would represent total masking or compensation for a sub-surface stromal cone and herald posterior elevation BFS changes which *do* represent keratoconus (Fig. 5). Conversely, finding thicker epithelium over an area of topographic steepening or an eccentric posterior elevation BFS apex would imply that the steepening is *not* due to a keratoconic sub-surface stromal cone but more likely due to localized epithelial thickening. Localized compensatory changes in epithelial thickness profiles can be

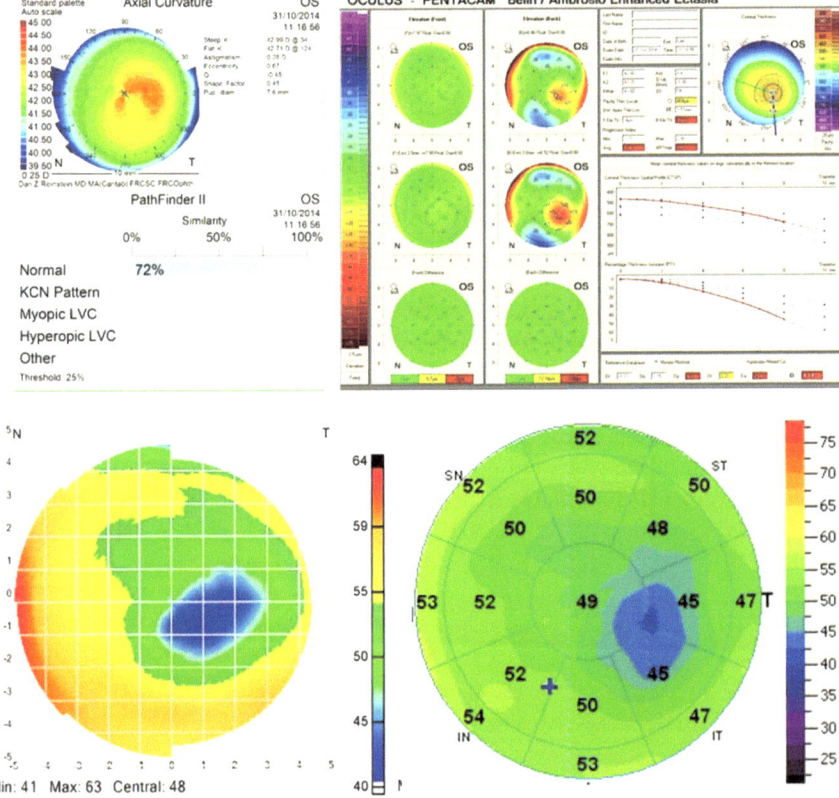

Fig. 5 Corneal epithelial maps (ArcScan Insight 100 and OptoVue RTVue) on the bottom row showing focal thinning, thus confirming the back surface elevation changes highlighted by Pentacam (top right) are indeed keratoconus. This is despite an Atlas topography map (top left) being inconclusive

detected by VHF digital ultrasound once they exceed 1–2 μm. In a way, examination of epithelial thickness profile irregularities provides a very sensitive method of examining stromal surface topography – by proxy. Therefore, this technique provides increased sensitivity and specificity to a diagnosis of keratoconus well in advance of any detectable corneal front surface topographic change.

Case Examples

Figure 4 shows three further selected examples where epithelial thickness profiles helped to interpret and diagnose anterior and posterior elevation BFS abnormalities. In each case, the epithelial thickness profile appears to be able to differentiate cases where the diagnosis of keratoconus is uncertain, from normal [78].

Case 1 (OS) represents a 25-year-old male, with a manifest refraction of -1.00 -0.50 × 150 and a best spectacle-corrected visual acuity of 20/16. Atlas corneal topography demonstrated inferior steepening which would traditionally indicate keratoconus. The keratometry was 45.25/43.25 D × 76, and PathFinder™ corneal analysis classified the topography as normal. Orbscan II posterior elevation BFS showed that the posterior elevation BFS apex was decentered inferotemporally. Corneal pachymetry minimum by handheld ultrasound was 479 μm. Contrast sensitivity was slightly below the normal range measured using the CSV-1000 (Vector Vision Inc., Greenville, Ohio). There was −0.30 μm (Optical Society (OSA) notation) of vertical coma on Wavefront Aberration Supported Corneal Ablation (WASCA) aberrometry. Corneal hysteresis was 7.5 mmHg, and corneal resistance factor was 7.1 mmHg, which are low, but these could be affected by the low corneal thickness. The combination of inferior steepening, an eccentric posterior elevation BFS apex, and thin cornea raised the suspicion of keratoconus although there was no suggestion of keratoconus by refraction, keratometry, or PathFinder™ corneal analysis. Artemis epithelial thickness profile showed a pattern typical of keratoconus with an epithelial doughnut shape characterized by a localized zone of epithelial thinning displaced inferotemporally over the eccentric posterior elevation BFS apex, surrounded by an annulus of thick epithelium. The coincidence of an area of epithelial thinning with the apex of the posterior elevation BFS, as well as the increased irregularity of the epithelium, confirmed the diagnosis of early keratoconus.

Case 2 (OD) represents a 31-year-old female, with a manifest refraction of -2.25 -0.50 × 88 and a best spectacle-corrected visual acuity of 20/16. Atlas corneal topography demonstrated a very similar pattern to case 1 of inferior steepening, therefore suggesting that the eye could also be keratoconic. The keratometry was 44.12/44.75 D × 148, and PathFinder™ corneal analysis classified the topography as suspect subclinical keratoconus. Orbscan II posterior elevation BFS showed that the apex was slightly decentered nasally. Corneal pachymetry minimum by handheld ultrasound was 538 μm. Contrast sensitivity was in the normal range. There was 0.32 μm (OSA notation) of vertical coma on WASCA aberrometry. Corneal hysteresis was 10.1 mmHg, and corneal resistance factor was 9.8 mmHg, which are well within normal range. The combination of inferior steepening, against-the-rule astigmatism, and high degree of vertical coma raised the suspicion of keratoconus, which was also noted by PathFinder™ corneal analysis. Artemis epithelial thickness profile showed a typical normal pattern with thicker epithelium inferiorly and thinner epithelium superiorly. Thicker epithelium inferiorly over the suspected cone (inferior steepening on topography) was inconsistent with an underlying stromal surface cone, and therefore the diagnosis of keratoconus was excluded. This patient would have been rejected for surgery given a documented PathFinder™ corneal analysis warning of suspect subclinical keratoconus, but given the epithelial thickness profile, this patient was deemed a suitable candidate for LASIK.

The anterior corneal topography in case 3 (OD) bears no features related to keratoconus. The patient is a 35-year-old female with a manifest refraction of -4.25 -0.50 × 4 and a best spectacle-corrected visual acuity of 20/16. The refraction had been stable for at least 10 years, and the contrast sensitivity was within normal limits. The keratometry was 43.62/42.62 D × 74, and PathFinder™ analysis classified the topography as normal. Orbscan II posterior elevation BFS showed that the apex was slightly decentered inferotemporally, but the anterior elevation BFS apex was well centered. Corneal pachymetry minimum by handheld ultrasound was 484 µm. Pentacam (Oculus, Wetzlar, Germany) keratoconus screening indices were normal. WASCA ocular higher-order aberrations were low (RMS = 0.19 µm) as well as the level of vertical coma (coma = 0.066 µm). Corneal hysteresis was 8.9 mmHg, and corneal resistance factor was 8.8 mmHg, both within normal limits. In this case, only the slightly eccentric posterior elevation BFS apex and the low-normal corneal thickness were suspicious for keratoconus, while all other screening methods gave no indication of keratoconus. However, the epithelial thickness profile showed an epithelial doughnut pattern characterized by localized epithelial thinning surrounded by an annulus of thick epithelium, coincident with the eccentric posterior elevation BFS apex. Epithelial thinning with surrounding annular thickening over the eccentric posterior elevation BFS apex indicated the presence of probable sub-surface keratoconus. In this case, it seems that the epithelium had fully compensated for the stromal surface irregularity so that the anterior surface topography of the cornea appeared perfectly regular. Given the regularity of the front surface topography and the normality of nearly all other screening parameters, it is feasible that this patient could have been deemed suitable for corneal refractive surgery and subsequently developed ectasia. As we were able to also consider the epithelial thickness profile, this patient was rejected for corneal refractive surgery. This kind of case may explain some reported cases of ectasia "without a cause" [79].

Automated Algorithm for Classification by Epithelium

Based on this qualitative diagnostic method, we set out to derive an automated classifier to detect keratoconus using epithelial thickness data, together with Ron Silverman and his group at Columbia University [80]. We used stepwise linear discriminant analysis (LDA) and neural network (NN) analysis to develop multivariate models based on combinations of 161 features comparing a population of 130 normal and 74 keratoconic eyes. This process resulted in a six-variable model that provided an area under the receiver operating curve of 100%, indicative of complete separation of keratoconic from normal corneas. Test-set performance, averaged over ten trials, gave a specificity of 99.5 ± 1.5% and sensitivity of 98.9 ± 1.9%. Maps of the average epithelium and LDA function values were also found to be well correlated with keratoconus severity grade (Figs. 6 and 7). Other groups have also been working on automated classification algorithms based on epithelial thickness data obtained by OCT [52, 81].

Following this study, we then applied the algorithm to a population of ten patients with unilateral keratoconus (clinically and algorithmically topographically normal in the fellow eyes), on the basis that the fellow eye in such patients represents a latent form of keratoconus and, as such, has been considered a gold standard for studies aimed at early keratoconus detection. These eyes were also analyzed using the Belin-Ambrosio enhanced ectasia display (BAD-D parameter and ART-Max) [20, 24, 82] and the Orbscan SCORE value as described by Saad and Gatinel [28–30].

Table 1 summarizes the diagnosis derived for the fellow eyes using the classification function based on epithelial thickness parameters, the classification function combining VHF digital ultrasound (epithelial and stromal thickness) and Pentacam HD parameters, the BAD-D and ART-Max values, and the Orbscan SCORE value. The last column of the table indicates whether the topographic map displayed suspicious features of keratoconus such as inferior steepening and asymmetric bow-tie. The table also shows the percentage of eyes that were classified as keratoconus by each method.

The most interesting finding of this study was that more than 50% of the fellow eyes were classified as normal by all methods. This was similar to the result reported

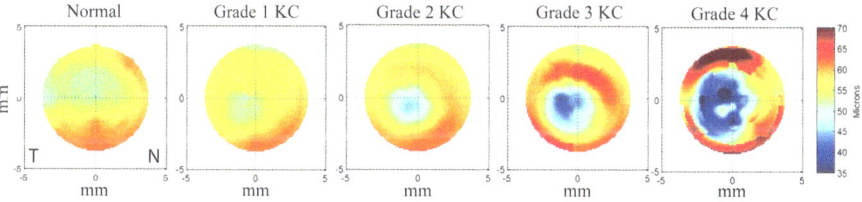

Fig. 6 Epithelial thickness maps averaged over all normal corneas and for each keratoconus grade. The departure from the normal epithelial distribution is evident even in grade 1 keratoconus but becomes more obvious with severity. (Reprinted with permission from IOVS: Silverman et al. [80])

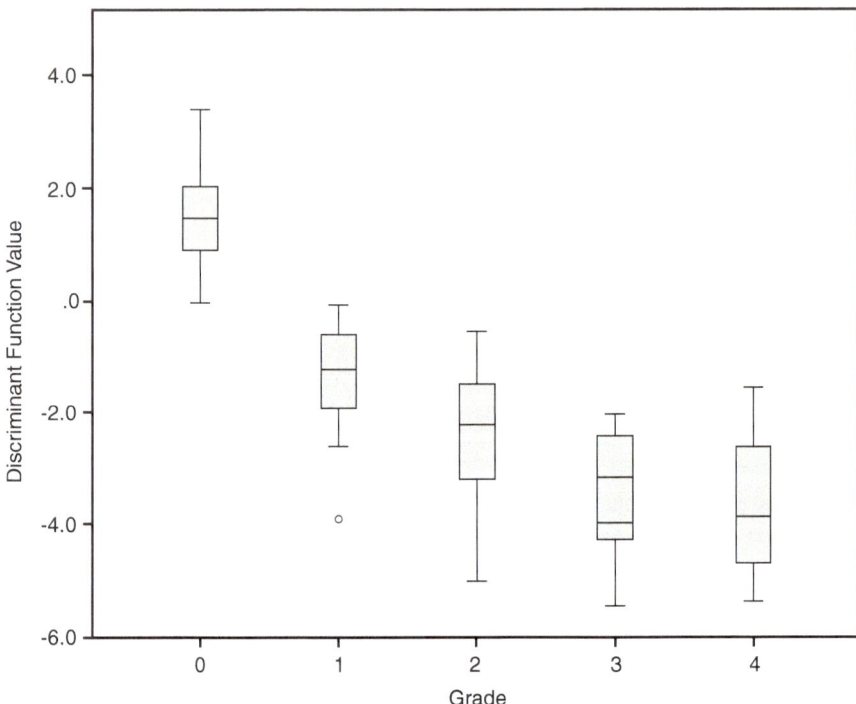

Fig. 7 Box and whisker plot of discriminant function value versus keratoconus severity grade. Grade 0 represents normal subjects. Grades 1–4 are based on Krumeich classification. Boxes represent ±1 quartile about median value (horizontal line), and whiskers represent full range of values for each group. Circles indicate outliers. (Reprinted with permission from IOVS: Silverman et al. [80])

by Bae et al. [26], who found no difference in the BAD-D or ART-Max values between normal and topographically normal fellow eyes of keratoconus patients. This is in contrast to other studies using unilateral keratoconic populations where a much higher sensitivity was reported; however, these studies often included patients with a suspicious topography in the fellow eye (i.e., some studies use a more rigorous definition of unilateral keratoconus than others) [27]. Therefore, the main conclusion from the study was to put into question the validity of using unilateral keratoconus patients for keratoconus screening studies. The fact that a number of these fellow eyes showed absolutely no indication of keratoconus by any method implies that it is likely that these were truly normal eyes. However, it is generally agreed that keratoconus as a disease must be bilateral [83]; therefore, it appears that these cases are patients who do not have keratoconus but have induced an ectasia in one eye, for example, by eye rubbing or trauma. This means that using "unilateral keratoconic" populations to study keratoconus screening may be flawed.

The alternative is somewhat more alarming, as this would mean that there are eyes with keratoconus that are literally undetectable by any existing method. This

Table 1 Keratoconus classification by four methods for ten fellow eyes classified as normal by topographic algorithm of patients with clinically evident unilateral keratoconus

Case	Classification function VHF digital only		Classification function VHF digital ultrasound + Pentacam HD		Pentacam HD				Orbscan II		Suspicious Atlas topographic features
	KC probability	Diagnosis	KC probability	Diagnosis	BAD-D	Diagnosis	ART-Max	Diagnosis	SCORE	Diagnosis	
1	69%	KC							−1.1	Normal	None
2	86%	KC							0.8	KC	None
3	94%	KC							−0.3	Normal	Skewed bow-tie Low astigmatism
4	4%	Normal							0.2	KC	None
5	83%	KC							5.6	KC	Asymmetric bow-tie Inferior steepening
6	<1%	Normal	<1%	Normal	−0.39	Normal	576	Normal			Small central bow-tie
7	<1%	Normal	<1%	Normal	0.83	Normal	454	Normal	−0.2	Normal	None
8	8%	Normal	95%	KC	1.35	Normal	380	Normal	0.6	KC	Asymmetric bow-tie Inferior steepening
9	76%	KC	12%	Normal	1.03	Normal	446	Normal	1.5	KC	None
10	<1%	Normal	<1%	Normal	0.07	Normal	524	Normal	−2.2	Normal	None
KC%		5/10 (50%)		1/5 (20%)		0/5 (0%)		0/5 (0%)		4/9 (55%)	
KC%		1/5 (20%)				0/5 (0%)		0/5 (0%)		2/5 (40%)	

First, predicted keratoconus probability and diagnostic category (classified as keratoconus probability was >50%) using the automated algorithm based on epithelial thickness data alone. Second, predicted keratoconus probability and diagnostic category (classified as keratoconus probability was >50%) using the automated algorithm based on epithelial thickness and corneal tomography data. Third, the BAD-D value taken from corneal tomography and the diagnostic category using a cutoff value of 1.45 to represent keratoconus. Fourth, the ART-Max value taken from corneal tomography and the diagnostic category using a cutoff value of 339 μm to represent keratoconus. Fifth, the SCORE algorithm value and the diagnostic category classified as keratoconus if >0 would, however, explain any case of "ectasia without a cause" [79, 84]. Detection of keratoconus in such cases may require development of new in vivo measurements of corneal biomechanics, although this appears to be outside the scope of current methods such as the ocular response analyzer [85–87] and Corvis (Oculus, Wetzlar, Germany) [86, 87] due to the wide scatter in the data acquired. Another factor, as has been described using Brillouin microscopy [88], may be that the biomechanical tensile strength of the cornea may not be different from normal in early keratoconus when measuring the whole cornea globally, but there may only be a difference in the region localized of the cone (or in the location of a future cone). Another potential and final solution would be whether a genotype or other molecular marker for keratoconus could be found [89–91].

Finally, another interpretation of this result is that keratoconus may not necessarily be a disease of abnormal stromal substance. The localization of the reduced corneal biomechanics found in keratoconus suggests that this may be caused by a local defect in Bowman's layer due to eye rubbing or other trauma. A break in Bowman's layer would reduce the tension locally, and the asymmetric stress concentration would then cause the stroma to bulge in this location. Evidence for changes in Bowman's layer in keratoconus has been reported using ultra-high-resolution OCT; Shousha et al. [92] showed that Bowman's layer was thinner inferiorly in keratoconus and described a Bowman's ectasia index (BEI) to be used for keratoconus screening. Yadav et al. [93] also described differences in the thickness of Bowman's layer in keratoconus, as well as a difference in light scatter.

Conclusion

Keratoconus detection is ever-evolving. We have demonstrated that the epithelial thickness profile was significantly different between normal eyes and keratoconic eyes. Whereas the epithelium in normal eyes was relatively homogeneous in thickness with a pattern of slightly thicker epithelium inferiorly than superiorly, the epithelium in keratoconic eyes was irregular showing a doughnut-shaped pattern and a marked difference in thickness between the thin epithelium at the center of the doughnut and the surrounding annulus of the thick epithelium. We have shown that the epithelial thickness profile progresses along with the evolution of keratoconus. More advanced keratoconus produces more irregularity in the epithelial thickness profile. We have found that the distinctive epithelial doughnut pattern associated with keratoconus can be used to confirm or exclude the presence of an underlying stromal surface cone in cases with normal or suspect front surface topography as well as can be a "qualifier" for the finding of an eccentric posterior elevation BFS apex.

Knowledge of the differences in epithelial thickness profile between the normal population and the keratoconic population allowed us to identify several features of the epithelial thickness profile that might help to discriminate between normal eyes and keratoconus-suspect eyes.

Randleman, in his paper assessing risk factors for ectasia, reported that ectasia might still occur after uncomplicated surgery in appropriately screened candidates [33]. Mapping of epithelial thickness profiles might provide an explanation for these cases; it could be that a stromal surface cone was masked by epithelial compensation and the front surface topography appeared normal.

Mapping of the epithelial thickness profile may increase sensitivity and specificity of screening for keratoconus compared to current conventional corneal topographic screening alone and may be useful in clinical practice in two very important ways.

Firstly, epithelial thickness mapping can exclude the appropriate patients by detecting keratoconus earlier or confirming keratoconus in cases where topographic changes may be clinically judged as being "within normal limits." Epithelial information allows an earlier diagnosis of keratoconus as epithelial changes will occur before changes on the front surface of the cornea become apparent. Epithelial thinning coincident with an eccentric posterior elevation BFS apex and in particular if surrounded by an annulus of thicker epithelium is consistent with keratoconus. Excluding early keratoconus patients from laser refractive surgery will reduce and potentially eliminate the risk of iatrogenic ectasia of this etiology and therefore increase the safety of laser refractive surgery. From our data, 136 eyes out of 1532 consecutive myopic eyes screened for refractive surgery demonstrated abnormal topography suspect of keratoconus. All 136 eyes were screened with Artemis VHF digital ultrasound arc-scanning, and individual epithelial thickness profiles were mapped. Out of 136 eyes with suspect keratoconus, only 22 eyes (16%) were confirmed as keratoconus [94].

Secondly, epithelial thickness profiles may be useful in excluding a diagnosis of keratoconus despite suspect topography. Epithelial thickening over an area of topographic steepening implies that the steepening is not due to an underlying ectatic surface. In such cases, excluding keratoconus using epithelial thickness profiles appears to allow patients who otherwise would have been denied treatment due to suspect topography to be deemed suitable for surgery. From our data, out of the 136 eyes with suspect keratoconus screened with Artemis VHF digital ultrasound arc-scanning, 114 eyes (84%) showed normal epithelial thickness profile and were diagnosed as non-keratoconic and deemed suitable for corneal refractive surgery. One-year post-LASIK follow-up data [94] and preliminary 2-year follow-up data [95] on these demonstrated equal stability and refractive outcomes as matched control eyes.

In summary, it is important to obtain a full clinical picture for the patient including demographic, diagnostic, and exam data. With advancements in keratoconus screening to include topography to tomography and now epithelium, we are seeing a shift in standard of care, and we are able to better serve our patients. In the future, advancements in algorithms and deep machine learning may prove to be yet another tool to aid in the early detection of keratoconus.

The contents of this chapter are summarized as a video lecture in Video 1.

Financial Disclosure Dr. Reinstein is a consultant for Carl Zeiss Meditec (Jena, Germany) and has a proprietary interest in the Artemis Technology (ArcScan Inc., Golden, Colorado) and is an author of patents related to VHF digital ultrasound administered by the Center for Technology Licensing at Cornell University, Ithaca, New York.

References

1. Ambrosio R Jr, Wilson SE. Complications of laser in situ keratomileusis: etiology, prevention, and treatment. J Refract Surg. 2001;17(3):350–79.
2. Seiler T, Koufala K, Richter G. Iatrogenic keratectasia after laser in situ keratomileusis. J Refract Surg. 1998;14(3):312–7.
3. Krachmer JH, Feder RF, Belin MW. Keratoconus and related non-inflammatory corneal thinning disorders. Surv Ophthalmol. 1984;28:293–322.
4. Wilson SE, Klyce SD. Screening for corneal topographic abnormalities before refractive surgery. Ophthalmology. 1994;101(1):147–52.
5. Klyce SD. Computer-assisted corneal topography. High-resolution graphic presentation and analysis of keratoscopy. Invest Ophthalmol Vis Sci. 1984;25(12):1426–35.
6. Rabinowitz YS, Yang H, Brickman Y, Akkina J, Riley C, Rotter JI, et al. Videokeratography database of normal human corneas. Br J Ophthalmol. 1996;80(7):610–6.
7. Rabinowitz YS, McDonnell PJ. Computer-assisted corneal topography in keratoconus. Refract Corneal Surg. 1989;5(6):400–8.
8. Rabinowitz YS. Videokeratographic indices to aid in screening for keratoconus. J Refract Surg. 1995;11(5):371–9.
9. Rabinowitz YS. Tangential vs sagittal videokeratographs in the "early" detection of keratoconus. Am J Ophthalmol. 1996;122(6):887–9.
10. Rabinowitz YS, Rasheed K. KISA% index: a quantitative videokeratography algorithm embodying minimal topographic criteria for diagnosing keratoconus. J Cataract Refract Surg. 1999;25(10):1327–35.
11. Smolek MK, Klyce SD. Current keratoconus detection methods compared with a neural network approach. Invest Ophthalmol Vis Sci. 1997;38(11):2290–9.
12. Maeda N, Klyce SD, Smolek MK. Comparison of methods for detecting keratoconus using videokeratography. Arch Ophthalmol. 1995;113(7):870–4.
13. Nesburn AB, Bahri S, Salz J, Rabinowitz YS, Maguen E, Hofbauer J, et al. Keratoconus detected by videokeratography in candidates for photorefractive keratectomy. J Refract Surg. 1995;11(3):194–201.
14. Chastang PJ, Borderie VM, Carvajal-Gonzalez S, Rostene W, Laroche L. Automated keratoconus detection using the EyeSys videokeratoscope. J Cataract Refract Surg. 2000;26(5):675–83.
15. Maeda N, Klyce SD, Smolek MK, Thompson HW. Automated keratoconus screening with corneal topography analysis. Invest Ophthalmol Vis Sci. 1994;35(6):2749–57.
16. Kalin NS, Maeda N, Klyce SD, Hargrave S, Wilson SE. Automated topographic screening for keratoconus in refractive surgery candidates. CLAO J. 1996;22(3):164–7.
17. Auffarth GU, Wang L, Volcker HE. Keratoconus evaluation using the Orbscan Topography System. J Cataract Refract Surg. 2000;26(2):222–8.
18. Rao SN, Raviv T, Majmudar PA, Epstein RJ. Role of Orbscan II in screening keratoconus suspects before refractive corneal surgery. Ophthalmology. 2002;109(9):1642–6.
19. Tomidokoro A, Oshika T, Amano S, Higaki S, Maeda N, Miyata K. Changes in anterior and posterior corneal curvatures in keratoconus. Ophthalmology. 2000;107(7):1328–32.
20. Ambrosio R Jr, Alonso RS, Luz A, Coca Velarde LG. Corneal-thickness spatial profile and corneal-volume distribution: tomographic indices to detect keratoconus. J Cataract Refract Surg. 2006;32(11):1851–9.

21. de Sanctis U, Loiacono C, Richiardi L, Turco D, Mutani B, Grignolo FM. Sensitivity and specificity of posterior corneal elevation measured by Pentacam in discriminating keratoconus/subclinical keratoconus. Ophthalmology. 2008;115(9):1534–9.
22. Saad A, Gatinel D. Evaluation of total and corneal wavefront high order aberrations for the detection of forme fruste keratoconus. Invest Ophthalmol Vis Sci. 2012;53(6):2978–92.
23. Luce DA. Determining in vivo biomechanical properties of the cornea with an ocular response analyzer. J Cataract Refract Surg. 2005;31(1):156–62.
24. Ambrosio R Jr, Caiado AL, Guerra FP, Louzada R, Roy AS, Luz A, et al. Novel pachymetric parameters based on corneal tomography for diagnosing keratoconus. J Refract Surg. 2011;27(10):753–8.
25. Fontes BM, Ambrosio R Jr, Salomao M, Velarde GC, Nose W. Biomechanical and tomographic analysis of unilateral keratoconus. J Refract Surg. 2010;26(9):677–81.
26. Bae GH, Kim JR, Kim CH, Lim DH, Chung ES, Chung TY. Corneal topographic and tomographic analysis of fellow eyes in unilateral keratoconus patients using Pentacam. Am J Ophthalmol. 2014;157(1):103–9. e1
27. Muftuoglu O, Ayar O, Ozulken K, Ozyol E, Akinci A. Posterior corneal elevation and back difference corneal elevation in diagnosing forme fruste keratoconus in the fellow eyes of unilateral keratoconus patients. J Cataract Refract Surg. 2013;39(9):1348–57.
28. Chan C, Ang M, Saad A, Chua D, Mejia M, Lim L, et al. Validation of an objective scoring system for forme fruste keratoconus detection and post-LASIK ectasia risk assessment in Asian eyes. Cornea. 2015;34(9):996–1004.
29. Saad A, Gatinel D. Validation of a new scoring system for the detection of early forme of keratoconus. Int J Kerat Ect Cor Dis. 2012;1(2):100–8.
30. Saad A, Gatinel D. Topographic and tomographic properties of forme fruste keratoconus corneas. Invest Ophthalmol Vis Sci. 2010;51(11):5546–55.
31. Mahmoud AM, Nunez MX, Blanco C, Koch DD, Wang L, Weikert MP, et al. Expanding the cone location and magnitude index to include corneal thickness and posterior surface information for the detection of keratoconus. Am J Ophthalmol. 2013;156(6):1102–11.
32. Randleman JB, Trattler WB, Stulting RD. Validation of the Ectasia Risk Score system for preoperative laser in situ keratomileusis screening. Am J Ophthalmol. 2008;145(5):813–8.
33. Randleman JB, Woodward M, Lynn MJ, Stulting RD. Risk assessment for ectasia after corneal refractive surgery. Ophthalmology. 2008;115(1):37–50.
34. Seiler T, Quurke AW. Iatrogenic keratectasia after LASIK in a case of forme fruste keratoconus. J Cataract Refract Surg. 1998;24(7):1007–9.
35. Speicher L, Gottinger W. Progressive corneal ectasia after laser in situ keratomileusis (LASIK). Klin Monatsbl Augenheilkd. 1998;213(4):247–51.
36. Geggel HS, Talley AR. Delayed onset keratectasia following laser in situ keratomileusis. J Cataract Refract Surg. 1999;25(4):582–6.
37. Amoils SP, Deist MB, Gous P, Amoils PM. Iatrogenic keratectasia after laser in situ keratomileusis for less than −4.0 to −7.0 diopters of myopia. J Cataract Refract Surg. 2000;26(7):967–77.
38. McLeod SD, Kisla TA, Caro NC, McMahon TT. Iatrogenic keratoconus: corneal ectasia following laser in situ keratomileusis for myopia. Arch Ophthalmol. 2000;118(2):282–4.
39. Holland SP, Srivannaboon S, Reinstein DZ. Avoiding serious corneal complications of laser assisted in situ keratomileusis and photorefractive keratectomy. Ophthalmology. 2000;107(4):640–52.
40. Schmitt-Bernard CF, Lesage C, Arnaud B. Keratectasia induced by laser in situ keratomileusis in keratoconus. J Refract Surg. 2000;16(3):368–70.
41. Rao SN, Epstein RJ. Early onset ectasia following laser in situ keratomileusus: case report and literature review. J Refract Surg. 2002;18(2):177–84.
42. Malecaze F, Coullet J, Calvas P, Fournie P, Arne JL, Brodaty C. Corneal ectasia after photorefractive keratectomy for low myopia. Ophthalmology. 2006;113(5):742–6.
43. Randleman JB, Russell B, Ward MA, Thompson KP, Stulting RD. Risk factors and prognosis for corneal ectasia after LASIK. Ophthalmology. 2003;110(2):267–75.

44. Leccisotti A. Corneal ectasia after photorefractive keratectomy. Graefes Arch Clin Exp Ophthalmol. 2007;245(6):869–75.
45. Reinstein DZ, Archer T. Combined Artemis very high-frequency digital ultrasound-assisted transepithelial phototherapeutic keratectomy and wavefront-guided treatment following multiple corneal refractive procedures. J Cataract Refract Surg. 2006;32(11):1870–6.
46. Reinstein DZ, Archer TJ, Gobbe M. Rate of change of curvature of the corneal stromal surface drives epithelial compensatory changes and remodeling. J Refract Surg. 2014;30(12):800–2.
47. Reinstein DZ, Silverman RH, Trokel SL, Coleman DJ. Corneal pachymetric topography. Ophthalmology. 1994;101(3):432–8.
48. Reinstein DZ, Silverman RH, Raevsky T, Simoni GJ, Lloyd HO, Najafi DJ, et al. Arc-scanning very high-frequency digital ultrasound for 3D pachymetric mapping of the corneal epithelium and stroma in laser in situ keratomileusis. J Refract Surg. 2000;16(4):414–30.
49. Reinstein DZ, Archer TJ, Gobbe M, Silverman RH, Coleman DJ. Epithelial thickness in the normal cornea: three-dimensional display with Artemis very high-frequency digital ultrasound. J Refract Surg. 2008;24(6):571–81.
50. Prakash G, Agarwal A, Mazhari AI, Chari M, Kumar DA, Kumar G, et al. Reliability and reproducibility of assessment of corneal epithelial thickness by fourier domain optical coherence tomography. Invest Ophthalmol Vis Sci. 2012;53(6):2580–5.
51. Ge L, Shen M, Tao A, Wang J, Dou G, Lu F. Automatic segmentation of the central epithelium imaged with three optical coherence tomography devices. Eye Contact Lens. 2012;38(3):150–7.
52. Li Y, Tan O, Brass R, Weiss JL, Huang D. Corneal epithelial thickness mapping by Fourier-domain optical coherence tomography in normal and keratoconic eyes. Ophthalmology. 2012;119(12):2425–33.
53. Reinstein DZ, Silverman RH, Coleman DJ. High-frequency ultrasound measurement of the thickness of the corneal epithelium. Refract Corneal Surg. 1993;9(5):385–7.
54. Bentivoglio AR, Bressman SB, Cassetta E, Carretta D, Tonali P, Albanese A. Analysis of blink rate patterns in normal subjects. Mov Disord. 1997;12(6):1028–34.
55. Doane MG. Interactions of eyelids and tears in corneal wetting and the dynamics of the normal human eyeblink. Am J Ophthalmol. 1980;89(4):507–16.
56. Young G, Hunt C, Covey M. Clinical evaluation of factors influencing toric soft contact lens fit. Optom Vis Sci. 2002;79(1):11–9.
57. Reinstein DZ, Gobbe M, Archer TJ, Couch D, Bloom B. Epithelial, stromal, and corneal pachymetry changes during orthokeratology. Optom Vis Sci. 2009;86(8):E1006–14.
58. Scroggs MW, Proia AD. Histopathological variation in keratoconus. Cornea. 1992;11(6):553–9.
59. Haque S, Simpson T, Jones L. Corneal and epithelial thickness in keratoconus: a comparison of ultrasonic pachymetry, Orbscan II, and optical coherence tomography. J Refract Surg. 2006;22(5):486–93.
60. Reinstein DZ, Archer TJ, Gobbe M, Silverman RH, Coleman DJ. Epithelial, stromal and corneal thickness in the keratoconic cornea: three-dimensional display with Artemis very high-frequency digital ultrasound. J Refract Surg. 2010;26(4):259–71.
61. Rocha KM, Perez-Straziota CE, Stulting RD, Randleman JB. SD-OCT analysis of regional epithelial thickness profiles in keratoconus, postoperative corneal ectasia, and normal eyes. J Refract Surg. 2013;29(3):173–9.
62. Kanellopoulos AJ, Aslanides IM, Asimellis G. Correlation between epithelial thickness in normal corneas, untreated ectatic corneas, and ectatic corneas previously treated with CXL; is overall epithelial thickness a very early ectasia prognostic factor? Clin Ophthalmol. 2012;6:789–800.
63. Sandali O, El Sanharawi M, Temstet C, Hamiche T, Galan A, Ghouali W, et al. Fourier-domain optical coherence tomography imaging in keratoconus: a corneal structural classification. Ophthalmology. 2013;120(12):2403–12.

64. Gauthier CA, Holden BA, Epstein D, Tengroth B, Fagerholm P, Hamberg-Nystrom H. Role of epithelial hyperplasia in regression following photorefractive keratectomy. Br J Ophthalmol. 1996;80(6):545–8.

65. Reinstein DZ, Srivannaboon S, Gobbe M, Archer TJ, Silverman RH, Sutton H, et al. Epithelial thickness profile changes induced by myopic LASIK as measured by Artemis very high-frequency digital ultrasound. J Refract Surg. 2009;25(5):444–50.

66. Reinstein DZ, Archer TJ, Gobbe M. Change in epithelial thickness profile 24 hours and longitudinally for 1 year after myopic LASIK: three-dimensional display with artemis very high-frequency digital ultrasound. J Refract Surg. 2012;28(3):195–201.

67. Kanellopoulos AJ, Asimellis G. Longitudinal postoperative lasik epithelial thickness profile changes in correlation with degree of myopia correction. J Refract Surg. 2014;30(3):166–71.

68. Reinstein DZ, Archer TJ, Gobbe M, Silverman RH, Coleman DJ. Epithelial thickness after hyperopic LASIK: three-dimensional display with artemis very high-frequency digital ultrasound. J Refract Surg. 2010;26(8):555–64.

69. Reinstein DZ, Archer TJ, Gobbe M. Epithelial thickness up to 26 years after radial keratotomy: three-dimensional display with artemis very high-frequency digital ultrasound. J Refract Surg. 2011;27(8):618–24.

70. Reinstein DZ, Srivannaboon S, Holland SP. Epithelial and stromal changes induced by intacs examined by three-dimensional very high-frequency digital ultrasound. J Refract Surg. 2001;17(3):310–8.

71. Reinstein DZ, Silverman RH, Sutton HF, Coleman DJ. Very high-frequency ultrasound corneal analysis identifies anatomic correlates of optical complications of lamellar refractive surgery: anatomic diagnosis in lamellar surgery. Ophthalmology. 1999;106(3):474–82.

72. Reinstein DZ, Archer TJ, Gobbe M. Refractive and topographic errors in topography-guided ablation produced by epithelial compensation predicted by three-dimensional Artemis very high-frequency digital ultrasound stromal and epithelial thickness mapping. J Refract Surg. 2012;28(9):657–63.

73. Reinstein DZ, Archer TJ, Gobbe M. Improved effectiveness of trans-epithelial phototherapeutic keratectomy versus topography-guided ablation degraded by epithelial compensation on irregular stromal surfaces [plus video]. J Refract Surg. 2013;29(8):526–33.

74. Reinstein DZ, Gobbe M, Archer TJ, Youssefi G, Sutton HF. Stromal surface topography-guided custom ablation as a repair tool for corneal irregular astigmatism. J Refract Surg. 2015;31(1):54–9.

75. Reinstein DZ, Archer TJ, Dickeson ZI, Gobbe M. Trans-epithelial phototherapeutic keratectomy protocol for treating irregular astigmatism based population on epithelial thickness measurements by Artemis very high-frequency digital ultrasound. J Refract Surg. 2014;30(6):380–7.

76. Reinstein DZ, Gobbe M, Archer TJ, Couch D. Epithelial thickness profile as a method to evaluate the effectiveness of collagen cross-linking treatment after corneal ectasia. J Refract Surg. 2011;27(5):356–63.

77. Vinciguerra P, Roberts CJ, Albe E, Romano MR, Mahmoud A, Trazza S, et al. Corneal curvature gradient map: a new corneal topography map to predict the corneal healing process. J Refract Surg. 2014;30(3):202–7.

78. Reinstein DZ, Archer TJ, Gobbe M. Corneal epithelial thickness profile in the diagnosis of keratoconus. J Refract Surg. 2009;25(7):604–10.

79. Klein SR, Epstein RJ, Randleman JB, Stulting RD. Corneal ectasia after laser in situ keratomileusis in patients without apparent preoperative risk factors. Cornea. 2006;25(4):388–403.

80. Silverman RH, Urs R, Roychoudhury A, Archer TJ, Gobbe M, Reinstein DZ. Epithelial remodeling as basis for machine-based identification of keratoconus. Invest Ophthalmol Vis Sci. 2014;55(3):1580–7.

81. Temstet C, Sandali O, Bouheraoua N, Hamiche T, Galan A, El Sanharawi M, et al. Corneal epithelial thickness mapping using Fourier-domain optical coherence tomography for detection of form fruste keratoconus. J Cataract Refract Surg. 2015;41(4):812–20.

82. Ambrosio R Jr, Faria-Correia F, Ramos I, Valbon BF, Lopes B, Jardim D, et al. Enhanced screening for ectasia susceptibility among refractive candidates: the role of corneal tomography and biomechanics. Curr Ophthalmol Rep. 2013;1(1):28–38.

83. Gomes JA, Tan D, Rapuano CJ, Belin MW, Ambrosio R Jr, Guell JL, et al. Global consensus on keratoconus and ectatic diseases. Cornea. 2015;34(4):359–69.

84. Ambrosio R Jr, Dawson DG, Salomao M, Guerra FP, Caiado AL, Belin MW. Corneal ectasia after LASIK despite low preoperative risk: tomographic and biomechanical findings in the unoperated, stable, fellow eye. J Refract Surg. 2010;26(11):906–11.

85. Reinstein DZ, Gobbe M, Archer TJ. Ocular biomechanics: measurement parameters and terminology. J Refract Surg. 2011;27(6):396–7.

86. Vellara HR, Patel DV. Biomechanical properties of the keratoconic cornea: a review. Clin Exp Optom. 2015;98(1):31–8.

87. Pinero DP, Alcon N. Corneal biomechanics: a review. Clin Exp Optom. 2014;40:991.

88. Scarcelli G, Besner S, Pineda R, Yun SH. Biomechanical characterization of keratoconus corneas ex vivo with Brillouin microscopy. Invest Ophthalmol Vis Sci. 2014;55(7):4490–5.

89. Abu-Amero KK, Al-Muammar AM, Kondkar AA. Genetics of keratoconus: where do we stand? J Ophthalmol. 2014;2014:641708.

90. Burdon KP, Vincent AL. Insights into keratoconus from a genetic perspective. Clin Exp Optom. 2013;96(2):146–54.

91. Rabinowitz YS, Dong L, Wistow G. Gene expression profile studies of human keratoconus cornea for NEIBank: a novel cornea-expressed gene and the absence of transcripts for aquaporin 5. Invest Ophthalmol Vis Sci. 2005;46(4):1239–46.

92. Abou Shousha M, Perez VL, Fraga Santini Canto AP, Vaddavalli PK, Sayyad FE, Cabot F, et al. The use of Bowman's layer vertical topographic thickness map in the diagnosis of keratoconus. Ophthalmology. 2014;121(5):988–93.

93. Yadav R, Kottaiyan R, Ahmad K, Yoon G. Epithelium and Bowman's layer thickness and light scatter in keratoconic cornea evaluated using ultrahigh resolution optical coherence tomography. J Biomed Opt. 2012;17(11):116010.

94. Reinstein DZ, Archer TJ, Gobbe M. Stability of LASIK in corneas with topographic suspect keratoconus, with keratoconus excluded by epithelial thickness mapping. J Refract Surg. 2009;25(7):569–77.

95. Reinstein DZ, Archer TJ, Gobbe M. Stability of LASIK in corneas with topographic suspect keratoconus confirmed non-keratoconic by epithelial thickness mapping: 2-years follow-up. San Fransisco: AAO; 2009.

Histopathological Findings in Keratoconus

Sabrina Bergeron, Bruno F. Fernandes, Patrick Logan, and Miguel N. Burnier Jr.

Histopathological Findings in Keratoconus

Keratoconus is a degenerative condition that is diagnosed clinically and is typically treated with rigid contact lens. Therefore, histopathological studies of keratoconus are limited to advanced cases where the diseased cornea is surgically removed and the patient receives a corneal graft. Nowadays, other corneal remodeling techniques are also available, providing an alternative option to corneal grafting [1].

On gross examination, keratoconic corneas are distorted into a pronounced conical shape. Figure 1 shows an enucleation specimen with advanced keratoconus, represented by a prominent conical deformation toward the central cornea (arrowhead). Also present in this specimen are retinal atrophy (asterisk) and vitreomacular traction (arrow); both are unrelated to keratoconus. In this particular specimen, the stromal thinning is pronounced in the periphery. Even though keratoconus is generally bilateral, the deformation is not always axial, nor is it symmetrical.

Following penetrating keratoplasty, a corneal button generally measuring 8 mm in diameter is obtained (Fig. 2). The button fixed in buffered formalin and representative sections are submitted for paraffin impregnation and routine histology processing. Cut sections are stained by hematoxylin and eosin (H&E) or with periodic acid-Schiff (PAS) to highlight basement membranes. Stained sections are then observed under a light microscope.

Histology of a normal cornea reveals five distinctive layers as depicted in Fig. 3: the epithelium, Bowman's layer, the stroma, Descemet's membrane, and the endothelium [2]. The epithelium is composed of five to seven layers of non-keratinized squamous epithelium that are attached to the basement membrane. Bowman's layer sits right under the epithelial basement membrane and consists of condensed

S. Bergeron (✉) · B. F. Fernandes · P. Logan · M. N. Burnier Jr.
The MUHC – McGill University Ocular Pathology & Translational Research Laboratory, Montreal, QC, Canada
e-mail: sabrina.bergeron@mail.mcgill.ca

© Springer Nature Switzerland AG 2021
C. Carriazo, M. J. Cosentino (eds.), *New Frontiers for the Treatment of Keratoconus*, https://doi.org/10.1007/978-3-030-66143-4_4

Fig. 1 Enucleation specimen showing a keratoconic cornea (arrowhead), areas of retinal atrophy (asterisk), and vitreomacular tractions (arrow)

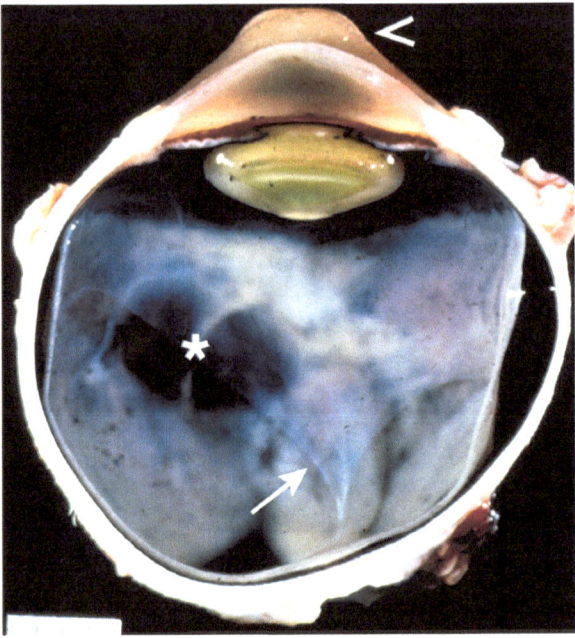

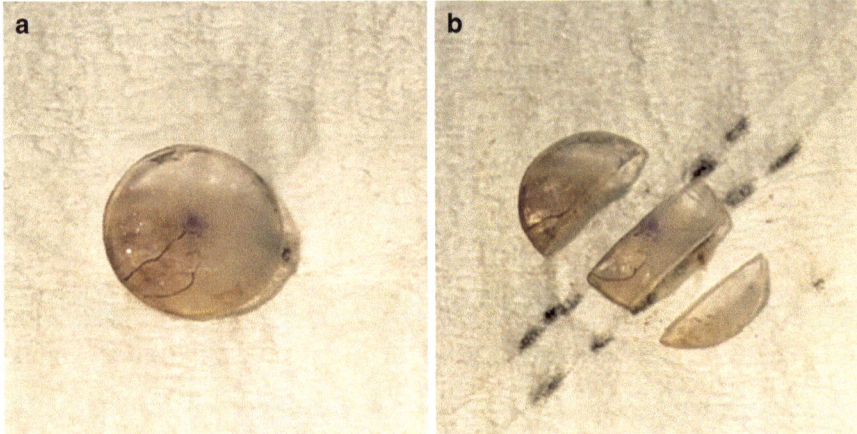

Fig. 2 Examples of a corneal button. (**a**) Corneal button with opacification and neovascularization (not keratoconus). (**b**) Representative sectioning of corneal button – the central portion is submitted for routine histopathological analysis

stromal fibers; it is acellular and is not a true membrane but a continuation of the corneal stroma. The corneal stroma is the thickest portion of the cornea, and it is represented by collagen fibers in a basket weave pattern. The stroma is responsible for most of the refractive power of the cornea, and its transparency is owed to active fluid transport out of the corneal stroma via the underlying endothelium. Descemet's

Fig. 3 Normal histological appearance of a human cornea: (I) epithelium, (II) basement membrane, (III) Bowman's layer, (IV) stroma, (V) Descemet's membrane, (VI) endothelium (PAS). (Image courtesy of Fernandes et al. [6])

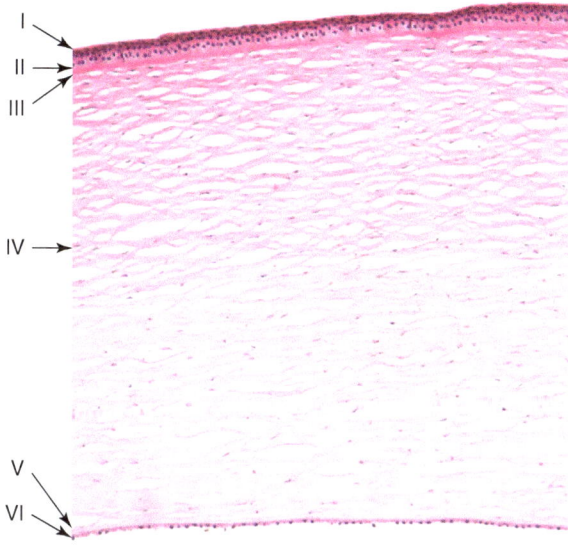

membrane is a true basement membrane composed of collagen and laminin, and it is produced by the endothelial cells. The endothelium is a monolayer of flattened cuboidal cells that appears as a honeycomb pattern if viewed from the posterior side. The endothelium is metabolically very active and maintains the cornea dry and transparent [2].

While the etiology and pathogenesis of keratoconus are still unknown, it is widely accepted that keratoconus is a disease of progressive and irregular thinning of the corneal tissue, leading to visual defects. The number of studies assessing histopathological findings in keratoconic corneas is limited [3–8], and there is a broad variety of different alterations that are reported in each corneal layer.

Two large series assessing histopathological findings of keratoconic corneas have been published, looking at 49 and 35 samples, respectively [5, 6]. In both studies, epithelial thinning was the most common histopathological feature (Fig. 4a), present in 87% of cases, and breaks in Bowman's layer (Fig. 4b) are observed in 76% of cases. Compaction of the stromal fiber (Fig. 4c) and folds or breaks in Descemet's membrane (Fig. 4d,e) are common, with a cumulative presence in 55% and 54% of cases, respectively. A superficial iron deposition in the epithelium (Fig. 4f) may also be observed, which is clinically seen as Fleischer's ring, but it is not required for the histopathological diagnosis of keratoconus.

It is suggested that epithelial thinning and the presence of breaks in Bowman's layer are related, which is referred to as typical keratoconus [3, 8]. Cases where Bowman's layer appears intact are usually referred to as atypical; however, they may also display marked epithelial thinning [3, 8]. A quantitative study of 36 keratoconic corneas shows an inverse correlation between the epithelial thickness and the number of breaks in Bowman's layer [3]. In that same study, authors gather evidence supporting two alternating patterns of epithelium: thinning and thickening

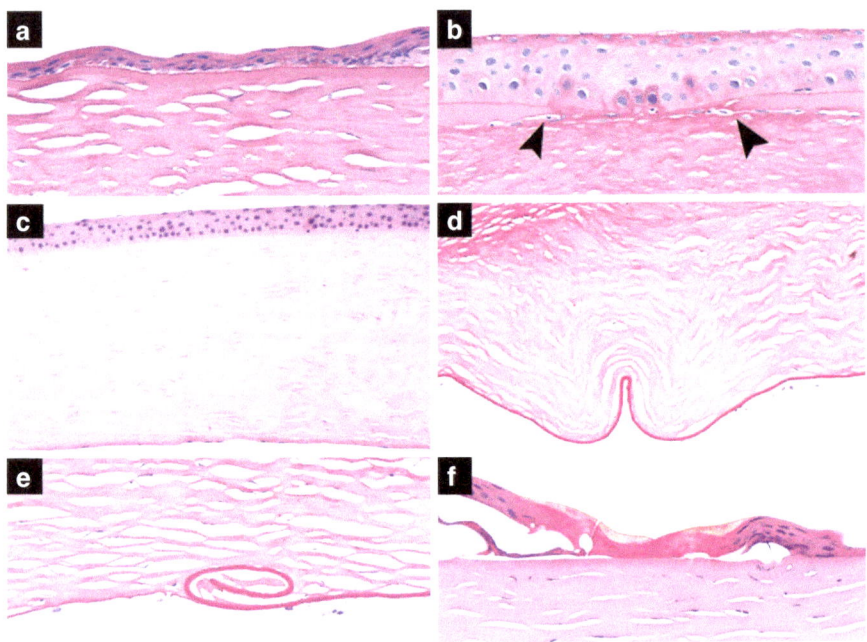

Fig. 4 Morphological changes in keratoconic corneas. (**a**) Epithelial thinning (PAS). (**b**) Break in Bowman's layer (between arrowheads) (PAS). (**c**) Compaction of stromal fibers (H&E). (**d**) Fold in Descemet's membrane (PAS). (**e**) Break in Descemet's membrane (PAS). (**f**) Iron deposits seen as a yellowish material overlying the epithelium (H&E). (Image courtesy of Fernandes et al. [6])

[3]. As both patterns can be observed within the same corneal sample, we conclude that keratoconic corneas display variable epithelial thickness.

The most commonly discussed histopathological aberrations of keratoconic corneas are located in the anterior cornea. Additionally, these anterior-most changes also correspond to the ones that can reliably be observed clinically by in vivo confocal microscopy [7]. However, the posterior portion of the cornea is also affected by the disease, most often in cases of advanced keratoconus. Stromal scarring is variably reported, and it is generally associated with stromal compaction, suggesting an end-stage disarrangement of the stromal structure [6]. Breaks and folds in Descemet's membrane are inconsistently reported across different studies, ranging from 18 to 63% [3, 5, 6]. It is hypothesized that alterations of Descemet's membrane are the result of environmental factors such as eye rubbing [9]. Some reports associate Descemet's rupture with cases of severe keratoconus and corneal hydrops [5].

Buffered formalin is a routinely used fixative in pathology. Alternatively, in a review of 12 corneas fixed in glutaraldehyde, the observations are comparable to formalin with the addition of a thickened basement membrane, a thinning epithelium, and a marked accumulation of cells and debris in the anterior stroma [4]. Data supporting this fixation protocol is limited, and others have observed a comparable opacification of the cornea whether they were fixed in glutaraldehyde or formalin

[10]. Further investigation is warranted in order to formulate recommendation on this noteworthy proposition.

Histopathological reviews of corneal buttons are generally limited to a number of representative sections. Therefore, a careful macroscopic description of the specimen is important in order to submit appropriate sections for processing and microscopic examination.

Although disruption in the stroma, Bowman's layer, or epithelium is pathognomonic of keratoconus, there is no histopathological finding that is seen in 100% of cases. A possible explanation is that keratoconus is a diagnosis based on clinical observations, and it is not impossible that different pathophysiological mechanisms are responsible for the changes associated with this particular disease.

In summary, explanted corneas with alterations of the whole thickness of the tissue are associated with advanced keratoconus [5]. Histopathological criteria for the diagnostic of keratoconus may include but are not limited to epithelial thinning, breaks in Bowman's layer, and stromal compaction.

References

1. Carriazo C, Cosentino MJ. A novel corneal remodeling technique for the management of keratoconus. J Refract Surg (Thorofare, NJ : 1995). 2017;33(12):854–6.
2. Forrester JV, Dick AD, McMenamin PG, Roberts F, Pearlman E. Chapter 1 – Anatomy of the eye and orbit. In: Forrester JV, Dick AD, McMenamin PG, Roberts F, Pearlman E, editors. The eye. 4th ed: W.B. Saunders; 2016. p. 1–102.e102.
3. Sykakis E, Carley F, Irion L, Denton J, Hillarby MC. An in depth analysis of histopathological characteristics found in keratoconus. Pathology. 2012;44(3):234–9.
4. Mathew JH, Goosey JD, Bergmanson JPG. Quantified histopathology of the keratoconic cornea. Optom Vis Sci. 2011;88(8):988–97.
5. Naderan M, Jahanrad A, Balali S. Histopathologic findings of keratoconus corneas underwent penetrating keratoplasty according to topographic measurements and keratoconus severity. Int J Ophthalmol. 2017;10(11):1640–6.
6. Fernandes BF, Logan P, Zajdenweber ME, Santos LN, Cheema DP, Burnier MN Jr. Histopathological study of 49 cases of keratoconus. Pathology. 2008;40(6):623–6.
7. Hollingsworth JG, Bonshek RE, Efron N. Correlation of the appearance of the keratoconic cornea in vivo by confocal microscopy and in vitro by light microscopy. Cornea. 2005;24(4):397–405.
8. Scroggs MW, Proia AD. Histopathological variation in keratoconus. Cornea. 1992;11(6):553–9.
9. Sherwin T, Brookes NH. Morphological changes in keratoconus: pathology or pathogenesis. Clin Exp Ophthalmol. 2004;32(2):211–7.
10. Moreira-Neto CA, Bergeron S, Coblentz J, et al. Optimizing optical coherence tomography and histopathology correlation in retinal imaging. Can J Ophthalmol: J canadien d'ophtalmologie. 2019;54(2):280–7.

Customized Corneal Cross-Linking

Theo G. Seiler

Theoretical Background

Today, the etiology of keratoconus is thought to be multifactorial [1]. Eye rubbing [2], in particular in atopy, genetic predisposition [3], and subclinical inflammations [4] are in discussion about the causes of keratoconus. As unilateral keratoconus seems to be a rare condition, it was also believed that if it is a genetic disease at all, it would affect the total cornea in both eyes. Also, it is known since decades that the keratoconus cornea is weaker than the normal cornea [5], and it is not clear why this weakness is limited to the cornea and does not impair other types of connective tissue.

A few years ago, a new approach came into discussion, mainly proposed by the Cleveland/Ohio group around Dupps and Roberts. They claimed that not the entire cornea needs to have a homogeneous reduction in stiffness but already a localized focal weakening of the cornea may induce a typical topographic keratoconus pattern. This idea was supported by finite-element simulations with a localized reduction of the elastic modulus of various degrees [6]. A focal weakening of the elastic modulus of the cornea by 10% had nearly no impact, but implying 30% and up to 45% resulted in a typical keratoconus shape. Although this idea was at first glance convincing, there were still some questions remaining: (1) the weakest point of the normal cornea is clearly the thinnest point which is in most cases in the center of the cornea. But why is in the majority of the keratoconus cases the bulging forward effect then localized inferior-temporally? (2) The assumption that the elastic

T. G. Seiler (✉)
Universitätsklinik für Augenheilkunde, Inselspital Bern, Bern, Switzerland

Wellman Center for Photomedicine – Massachusetts General Hospital, Harvard Medical School, Boston, MA, USA

Institut für Refraktive und Ophthalmo-Chirurgie (IROC), Zürich, Switzerland
e-mail: theo@seiler.tv

© Springer Nature Switzerland AG 2021
C. Carriazo, M. J. Cosentino (eds.), *New Frontiers for the Treatment of Keratoconus*, https://doi.org/10.1007/978-3-030-66143-4_5

modulus is focally reduced is not very reasonable because the turnover of the cornea is mediated by keratocytes and the distribution of the keratocytes is homogeneous.

Most of our doubts were overruled by Brillouin spectroscopy measurements in keratoconus corneas [7, 8]. Brillouin spectroscopy measures the bulk modulus M of a cornea which is different from the well-known elastic modulus E that represents the surface-parallel component of the elastic tensor. Although measuring not our usual elasticity of the cornea, this bulk modulus M represents a measure for stiffness, and we and others demonstrated that the bulk modulus was significantly reduced in the cone compared to the non-ectatic area [7, 8]. So it is not only the thinning that makes the cornea locally weak, but also the elastic moduli decrease in the cone region which can be interpreted as focal weakening of the cornea.

Considering these findings, the idea came up to strengthen only in this weak part of the cornea in order to reduce the lateral biomechanical gradient with potential benefits in shape regularization.

Technical Requirements and Limitations

If we want to treat only the weak part of the keratoconus cornea, we first need to identify which area is affected: is it the area around the point of K-max, the thinnest point, or the locus of the maximal posterior elevation?

Recently, we had the opportunity to compare Brillouin stiffness maps to geometrical Scheimpflug maps in a larger series or keratoconus eyes. The case shown in Fig. 1 with iatrogenic keratectasia after LASIK and progressive inferior steepening illustrates the difference of these three points. Here the distance between the thinnest point, the point of K_{max}, and the point of maximal float is more than 2 mm. The answer of this question for the weakest point was, again, answered by Brillouin spectroscopy which was performed in a clinical environment at IROC in Zürich, in 2017 [8]. Brillouin spectroscopy defined the weakest point clearly close to the maximum of the posterior elevation (Fig. 1). This decision is also plausible because the epithelium modulates and regularizes the anterior surface by the XYZ strategy: epithelial thickness is greater over areas of flattening and is thinner over steep areas.

The next questions that had to be answered was the areal distribution of the ultraviolet radiation assuming that we had homogeneous riboflavin distribution. For standard keratoconus, we decided to use concentric circular or elliptical areas with diameters depending on the dimensions of posterior elevation map ranging from 2 to 7 mm. The common center of the three circles was located over the maximum of the posterior float.

Although some studies used 15 J/cm^2 as the total radiant exposure, we perform customized CXL with an upper limit of 10 J/cm^2. The reason is a recommendation of the committee for the safety of non-ionizing radiation of the European community [9] that reported an upper limit of such radiation at 360 nm to be 1 J/cm^2 to

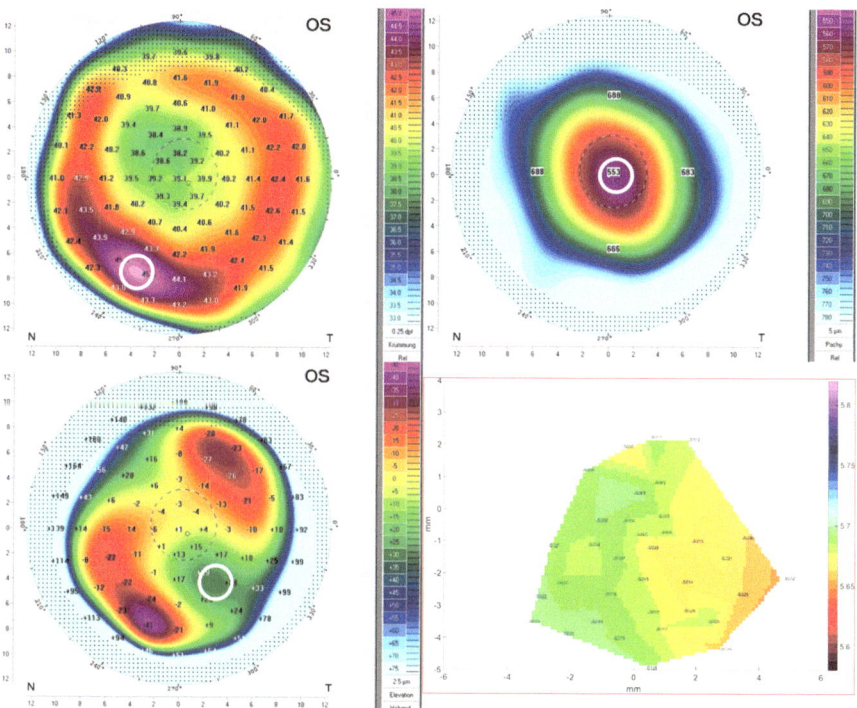

Fig. 1 Anterior sagittal curvature (top left), pachymetry (top right), posterior elevation map (reference body: best-fit sphere of the inner 8 mm) (bottom left), and Brillouin frequency shift map (bottom right) of a patient suffering from a progressive iatrogenic post-LASIK ectasia. White circles are indicating the maxima of each map. The maximal posterior elevation has the best overlap with the weakest point (lowest modulus, orange) obtained from Brillouin spectroscopy

prevent thermal cataractogenesis. From earlier experiments, we know that approximately 90% of the 360 nm radiation is absorbed by the riboflavin in a saturated cornea [10, 11], so that we can go up to 10 J/cm^2 as maximal radiant exposure.

It is well known from several publications that the efficiency of the cross-linking decreases with increasing irradiances [12, 13]. Therefore, we recommend using irradiances not greater than 18 mW/cm^2. As a consequence, the completion of full irradiation pattern in customized cross-linking may take up to 30 minutes, which makes an eye-tracking device mandatory.

The Avedro System Mosaic fulfills all these requirements, and the location of the centers of the irradiation areas can be imported digitally from Pentacam U12 files.

The surgical part consists of a manual epithelial debridement within the irradiation zone followed by the imbibition using 0.1% riboflavin with 1.1% hydroxypropylmethylcellulose (HPMC) for 10 minutes or 30 minutes, if 20% dextran is used as the osmotic agent [14]. When a sufficient corneal pachymetry is assured (>400 microns), the irradiation using the predesigned pattern can be initiated.

Clinical Experience

In the international literature, there are currently four publications on customized cross-linking with the first results published in 2016 [15] and three more articles that confirmed the original results in 2017 [16–18]. All studies used a prospective design comparing results of customized CXL with standard CXL according to the Dresden protocol. The first clinical benefit derived by customization of the procedure is a shorter epithelial healing time, resulting in a safety improvement because the vulnerable phase for infections and melting is shortened. Our group reported an average time until the closure of the epithelium of 2.6 days after customized CXL compared to 3.2 days after standard CXL. Similar to standard CXL, demarcation lines are also visible 1 month after customized CXL in the majority of the treated eyes. But in contrast to standard CXL, demarcation lines after customized CXL were not surface-parallel but showed a "Gaussian profile": deep in cone area and more shallow toward the peripheral, non-ectatic part of the cornea as depicted in Fig. 2. During the first postoperative year, the Toulouse study group [17] analyzed corneal nerve density and keratocyte apoptosis by means of confocal microscopy. A significant lower apoptosis rate is reported outside the cone as well as a higher nerve density. This might serve as another good reason why patients who experienced

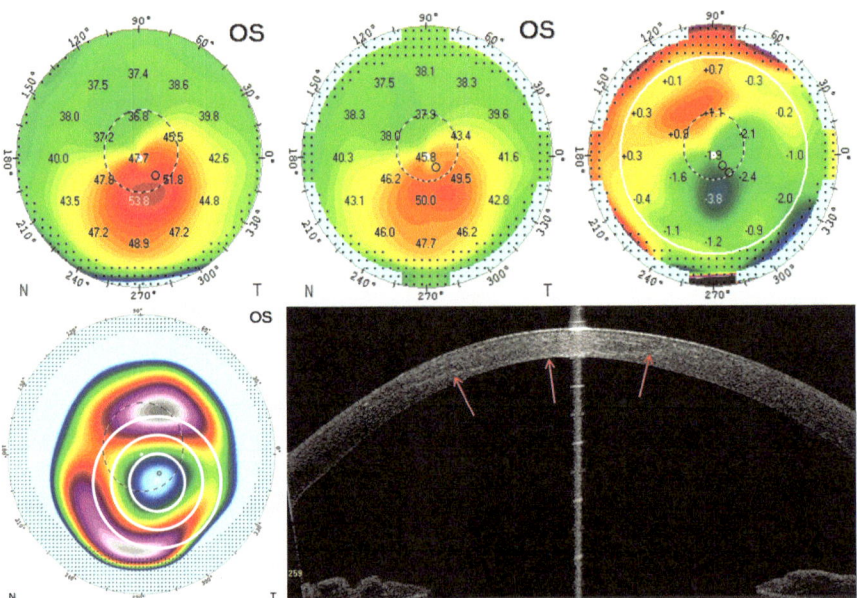

Fig. 2 Typical evolution of a patient treated with customized corneal cross-linking Preoperative sagittal curvature (top left), sagittal curvature at the 12-month follow-up (top middle), difference map (top right), preoperative posterior elevation map and the irradiation pattern (bottom left), and demarcation line at the 1-month follow-up emphasized with arrows (bottom right). ΔK_{max} is 3.6 diopters (D); regularization index (RI) is 5.3 D

both procedures describe the customized treatment as more comfortable. Topographical results after 1 year show a superior behavior of customized CXL over standard CXL. A typical case is depicted in Fig. 2. K_{max} and also K_{steep} experienced a significantly higher reduction after customized CXL compared to standard CXL with average regression rates of K_{max} of -1.7 D in customized CXL. When analyzing the distribution of flattening after both procedures, a flattening of ≥ 1 D is observed in 40% of eyes treated with standard CXL and in 60% of eyes treated with customized CXL. This increase by 50% is remarkable. However, not only the ratio of patients experiencing a flattening is increased, but also the chance of achieving strong flattening is increased. In standard CXL, only 10% of the treated eyes flatten by ≥ 3 D, whereas in customized CXL, this strong flattening is observed in more than 20% of eyes treated. When looking at 3-year follow-up data, a further increase in average flattening is observed; however, larger confirmation studies are needed.

The combination of customized cross-linking with a 100% oxygen environment is the latest development and currently under investigation in prospective studies. The higher oxygen availability is heralded to enable a more efficient superficial cross-linking process yielding higher stiffening rates. Preliminary, unpublished 4-month prospective data from the University of Bern looks promising with drastically enhanced flattening rates.

It is not only the flattening that makes the shape of the keratoconus cornea better, but parallel to the flattening, a steepening of the originally flat areas may occur (Fig. 2). This results in a regularization of the highly aberrated keratoconus cornea, and, therefore, a regularization index was coined that includes the flattening and the steepening effect [15]. This regularization index was better after customized CXL compared to standard CXL.

The active eye tracker guarantees protection of the limbal stem cells from accidental UV irradiation in customized CXL. This enables more precise and safer peripheral irradiations, which is, in particular for pellucid marginal degeneration, a big advantage. However, due to the higher radiant exposures of up to 15 J/cm², the risk for focal endothelial damage might be increased. Since endothelial damage is a severe complication, this needs to be addressed specifically. Although profound demarcation lines of up to 95% depth (Fig. 2) can be observed in customized CXL, no endothelial cell count reduction has been reported in any study until today [15–18]. A possible explanation might be the substantially lower riboflavin concentration within Descemet's membrane and the endothelium of less than 0.02% when using a 10-minute imbibition, which has been recently investigated by two-photon fluorescence microscopy [19]. On the other hand, no borderline cross-linking of corneas with a thinnest pachymetry of less than 400 microns prior to the UV irradiation has been performed/reported yet.

In summary, customization of CXL increases the safety of the procedure and enhances the outcome resulting in higher qualitative and quantitative flattening. Although the 1-year results are promising for the treatment of keratoconus, longer follow-up with larger numbers of treated eyes is not yet available, and a final assessment of the procedure can currently not be made. A promising further development might be the use of supplementary oxygen during customized CXL.

References

1. Krachmer JH. Eye rubbing can cause keratoconus. Cornea. 2004;23:539–40.
2. Sugar J, Macsai MS. What causes keratoconus? Cornea. 2012;31:716–9.
3. Valgaeren H, Koppen C, Van Camp G. A new perspective on the genetics of keratoconus: why have we not been more successful? Ophthalmic Genet. 2017;7:1–17.
4. Galvis V, Sherwin T, Tello A, et al. Keratoconus: an inflammatory disorder? Eye (Lond). 2015;29:843–59.
5. Andreassen TT, Simonsen AH, Oxlund H. Biomechanical properties of keratoconus and normal corneas. Exp Eye Res. 1980;4:435–51.
6. Roberts CJ, Dupps WJ Jr. Biomechanics of corneal ectasia and biomechanical treatments. J Cataract Refract Surg. 2014;40:991–8.
7. Scarcelli G, Besner S, Pineda R, et al. Biomechanical characterization of keratoconus corneas ex vivo with Brillouin microscopy. Invest Ophthalmol Vis Sci. 2014;55:4490–5.
8. Seiler TG, Shao P, Eltony A, Seiler T, Yun SH. Brillouin spectroscopy of normal and keratoconus corneas. Am J Ophthalmol. 2019 Jun;202:118–25.
9. The International Commission on Non-Ionizing Radiation Protection. ICNIRP Guidelines on Limits of Exposure to Laser Radiation of Wavelengths between 180 nm and 1,000 μm. Health Phys. 2013;105(3):271–95.
10. Seiler TG, Fischinger I, Senfft T, Schmidinger G, Seiler T. Intrastromal application of riboflavin for corneal crosslinking. Invest Ophthalmol Vis Sci. 2014;55:4261–5.
11. Koppen C, Gobin L, Tassignon MJ. The absorption characteristics of the human cornea in ultraviolet-a crosslinking. Eye Contact Lens. 2010;36:77–80.
12. Hammer A, Richoz O, Arba Mosquera S, et al. Corneal biomechanical properties at different corneal cross-linking (CXL) irradiances. Invest Ophthalmol Vis Sci. 2014;55:2881–1884.
13. Wernli J, Schumacher S, Spoerl E, et al. The efficacy of corneal cross-linking shows a sudden decrease with very high intensity UV light and short treatment time. Invest Ophthalmol Vis Sci. 2013;54:1176–80.
14. Ehmke T, Seiler TG, Fischinger I, et al. Comparison of corneal riboflavin gradients using dextran and HPMC solutions. J Refract Surg. 2016;32:798–802.
15. Seiler TG, Fischinger I, Koller T, et al. Customized corneal cross-linking: one-year results. Am J Ophthalmol. 2016;166:14–21.
16. Nordström M, Schiller M, Fredriksson A, et al. Refractive improvements and safety with topography-guided corneal crosslinking for keratoconus: 1-year results. Br J Ophthalmol. 2017;101:920–5.
17. Cassagne M, Pierné K, Galiacy SD, et al. Customized topography-guided corneal collagen cross-linking for keratoconus. J Refract Surg. 2017;33:290–7.
18. Shetty R, Pahuja N, Roshan T, et al. Customized corneal cross-linking using different UVA beam profiles. J Refract Surg. 2017;33:676–82.
19. Seiler TG, Batista A, Frueh BE, Koenig K. Riboflavin concentrations at the endothelium during corneal cross-linking in humans. Invest Ophthalmol Vis Sci. 2019;60:2140–5.

An Essential Guide to Treat Primary Ectasia with Intracorneal Segments

Roberto Gustavo Albertazzi

Basic Concepts of Additive Surgery

Additive surgery (addition: the act or process of adding) is a type of refractive surgery in which grafts or tissues are implanted around the visual axis without interfering directly with it. If the placement of materials is performed within the visual axis, then it would imply, for example, the placement of an intraocular lens of which the predictability of their effect is very high due to their design and location.

Additive surgery offers the advantage of reinforcing the tissue where the implants are added as it enhances structures with different variations of materials and designs. However, there is a lack of predictability with regard to its effects due to different parameters such as corneal elasticity, pachymetry, keratometry, and the diameter where the implants are placed, as well as their profiles and volumes should also be taken into account.

All these variables increase the possibility of intervening on corneal tissues with and without preserved function and structure. Moreover, the use of FemtoLaser makes it possible to treat not only ectasias but also corneal asymmetries that are yet to be confirmed as normal.

The basis of the indications started when the FDA approved the Intacs intracorneal implants for myopia [1]. Consequently, the appearance of the flat segments of Ferrara, the different arches, the change of optical zone to 6 mm, the asymmetric segments, and the combination of these profiles offered an unthinkable therapeutic range in only few years.

This chapter is divided into the following sections:

Intracorneal Segments
- Anatomy
- Models in the market

R. G. Albertazzi (✉)
Cornea and Refractive Surgery, Quilmes, Argentina

© Springer Nature Switzerland AG 2021
C. Carriazo, M. J. Cosentino (eds.), *New Frontiers for the Treatment of Keratoconus*, https://doi.org/10.1007/978-3-030-66143-4_6

- Effects on the corneal tissue depending on its design

Corneal Ectasia
- Classification by origin and structural behavior
- Most frequent patterns in primary ectasias

  Stage, behavior, and selection of segments to be implanted

- The best strategies to be chosen for each pattern

Anatomy of Intracorneal Rings Segments (ICRS)

It is essential to know from the very beginning the materials and supplies with which we are going to work. We shall start with the description below.

In Fig. 1, the most important characteristics of the segments are described.

Material

The material used for manufacturing the segments can be found in plastics such as polymethyl methacrylate, also known as PMMA [1].

The material used for the segments is PMMA – Perspex QC – which absorbs UV radiation and is manufactured according to the FDA, ISO 9001, and EN46001 requirements [1].

Apical Diameter

The apical diameter (Fig. 1) is determined by the line that crosses the center of the body of the segments so as to mark the diameter of the optical zone that they enclose; the said segments may be 5 mm, 6 mm, 7 mm of optical zone. Although it may not be the real central optical zone, this system simplifies the classification of the diameter of the segments.

Base

The base is the side on which the segment is placed (Fig. 1) and it is always toward the corneal endothelium, leaving its main base in the depth of the stroma. The different bases are related to the diameter and the profile and they are absolutely important in the final effect of the implant, since the base is the one that shows the profile of the segment with its angle.

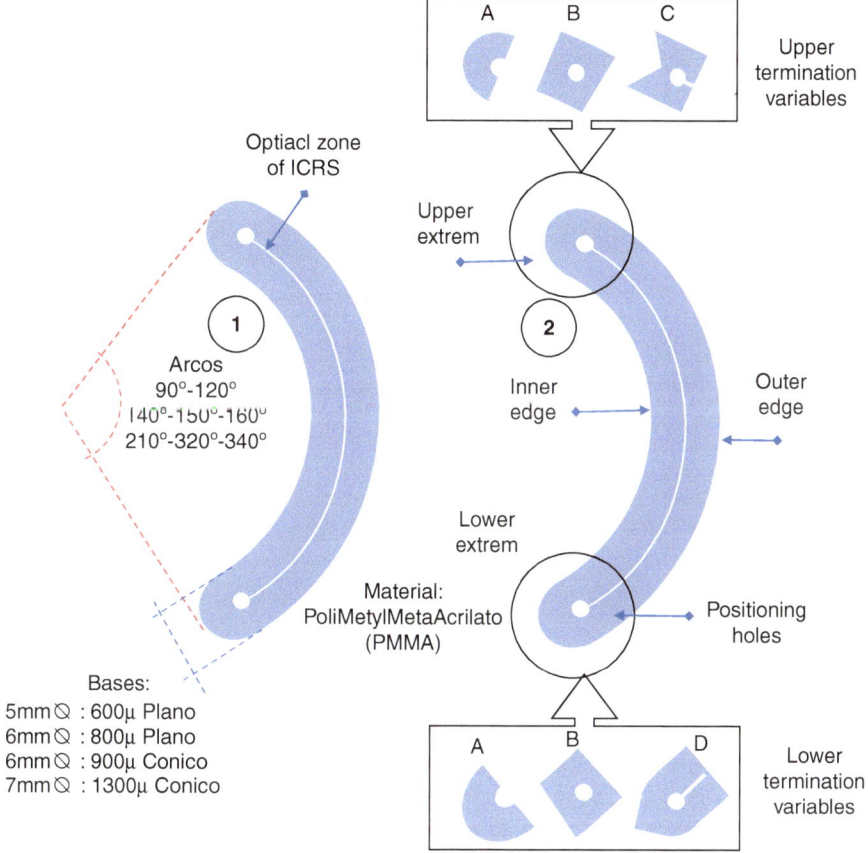

Fig. 1 (1) Apical diameter – short, medium, and long arcs. Different bases are according to the diameter and profile. (2) Upper variables of the ends – inner edge; lower variables of the ends – external edge

The old 5-mm diameter segments with a flat base need 600 microns to achieve their effect, while the conical segments with a diameter of 7 mm need up to 1330 microns at their base in order to generate an effect. The most frequently used segments are shown in Fig. 2.

Measures: Millimeters vs Microns

Some segment manufacturers use millimeters to identify the characteristics of their implants (Ferrara Ring), but refractive surgeons are used to working with microns (µ). One millimeter is equivalent to 100 microns, in other words 0.25 mm is equal to 250 microns.

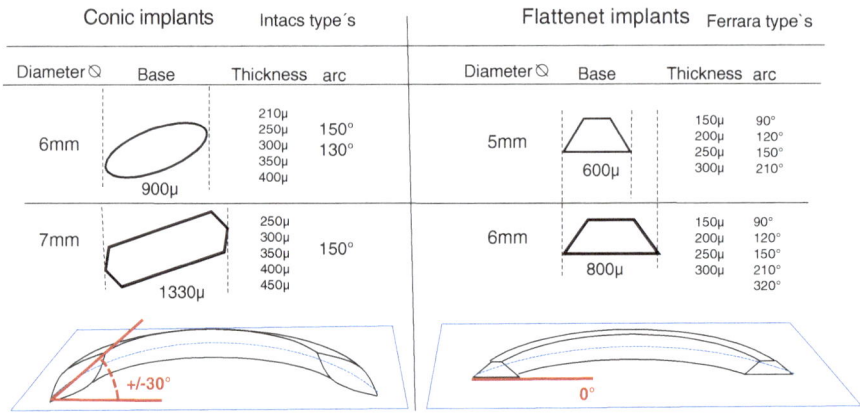

Fig. 2 Left: Conica Intac's Type base segments pointing to diameter, base, thicknesses, and arcs. Down: Graphing on a plane of the ± 30 degrees angle that they present. Right: Ferrara's type flat base segments pointing to diameter, base, thicknesses, and arches. Down: Graphing on a plane of the 0th angle that they present

Section

There are two sections: profiles or the tilts of the segments.

Flat segment (Ferrara type) which means 0° is a flat implant that is hard to implant within a conic structure due to the tension it generates in the structure where it is kept because the flat segment and the conic cornea have different designs (Fig. 2). This tension generates a reduction in the K values, which is just above the body of the segment, and an elevation of the tissue between the extremes, thanks to the release of the tension vectors they generate. These flat segments, originally designed by Ferrara and manufactured by several companies (Ferrara Rings®, Easy Ring®, Keraring ® Mediphacos®, Intraseg®, etc.), have a flat base as their design which must be parallel to the corneal endothelium and without any type of angle.

Conic section segments (Intacts type) keep a tilt of about 26–34° of their base that may have different angles as regard tilting (12°, 17°, 32°, or 34°) according to the manufacturer (Fig. 2). These designs are similar to the corneal curvature and do not oppose to it, making them much easier to insert. Additionally, they hardly generate intracorneal tension and cause their effect by increasing the volume of the tissue. This is why the conic segments keep their corneal prolaticity without generating new astigmatisms.

External Edge

The implanted material must respect a free space to the limbo. Otherwise, the growth of blood vessels can be stimulated due to its proximity. Some time ago, I discovered that if flat segments were introduced in the channel, they slid more easily

Fig. 3 Left: External edge modifications introduced by the author (Abertazzi R) transforming them into injectables; right: different types of injectors (USA N° 29/649, 370/344)

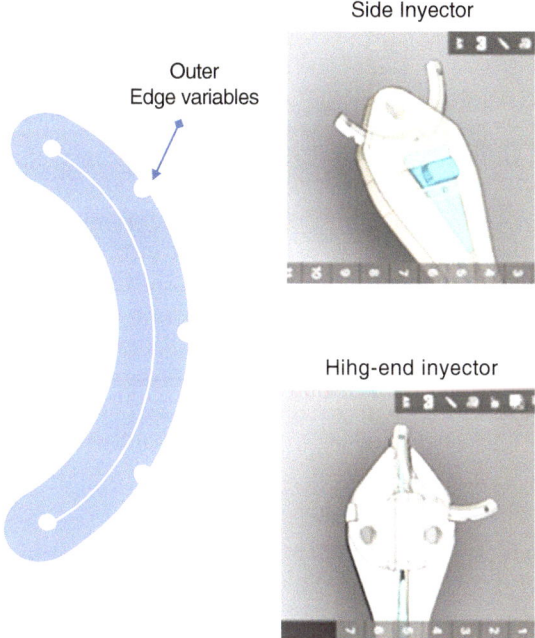

Outer
Edge variables

Side Inyector

Hihg-end inyector

when manipulated from the edge. Taking this into account, I managed to develop the injectable segments [2] by making some small low notches on the edge (Fig. 3).

Inner Edge

The inner edge marks the area of the optical zone, so the centering of the smallest segments (5 mm optical zone) must be strict. Otherwise, glare symptoms could appear if they are a bit off-centered (Fig. 1–2).

Currently, 6-mm diameter segments are used (in almost 100% of the cases), leaving the use of 5- mm diameter segments for special cases such as post corneal-graft high astigmatism or asymmetry.

Ends

For years, nobody paid attention to the ends (Fig. 1), being usually round in the case of the Ferrara and flat in the Intacts.

The first change made to the ends took place with the appearance of the asymmetric segments, where the distal end was designed with a pointed shape and the proximal end with a low notch (Figs. 1 and 7). The correct way to insert them was pointed outward. The widest end was at the distal point and the narrowest at the proximal end.

Thickness

With regard to the thickness of the implants, it was Blavastskaya who first described the direct relationship between the effect and the thickness, which implied that the bigger the implant thickness is, the stronger the effect.

It is to be highlighted that Blavastskaya [3] carried out his study using stromal corneal implants, which are soft, compressible and flexible, and different from the stiffness of the PMMA which is currently used. Therefore, although there is a law, and only to some extent, the behaviors of the stroma (viscoelasticity and compressibility) have nothing to do with the stiffness of the PMMA.

Effects of the Different Segments Within the Corneal Stroma

Figure 4a shows how a conic-shaped segment schematically makes contact with an ellipsoid shape, represented by a balloon, whereas (b) shows the contact it makes with a flat segment. It may be easy to imagine that a conical segment will show less

Profile

a Conic (Intacs type´s)   **b**   Flattenet (Ferrara type´s)

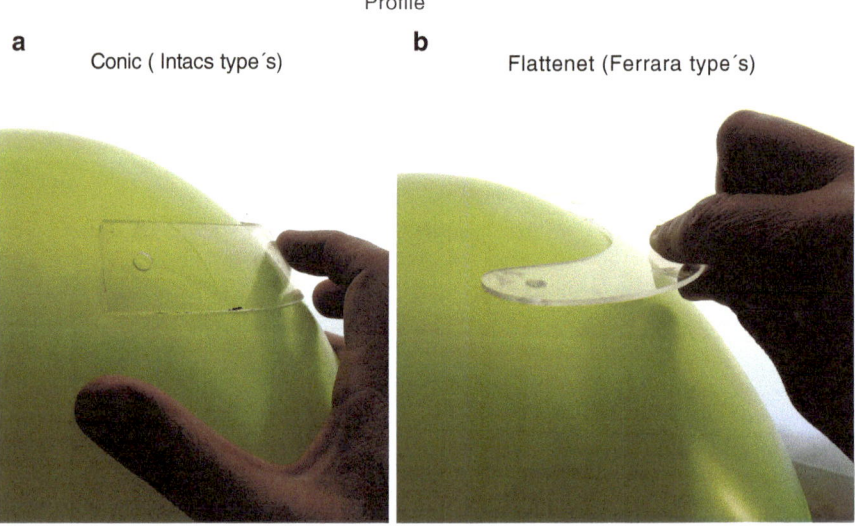

Fig. 4 (**a**) Conic type's ICRS and Ferrara type's ICRS make contact resulting in an ellipsoid shape, like balloon

resistance as it is part of an ellipsoid, represented by the balloon. However, it is hard to imagine the flat segment being part of it.

In Fig. 5a, to the left, we can observe a presurgical spherical topography of two 150° 6-mm diameter arch conical segments (represented in the center). On the right, the effect they produce once they are implanted can be seen. It is clearly observed that the corneal structure keeps its own prolaticity, inherent to it, despite having less keratometric values, and does not generate astigmatisms.

Figure 6 shows the flat segments that are placed in a spherical cornea, producing astigmatism (a). If we place them in an astigmatic cornea (such as an ectasia), the preexisting astigmatism is reduced or corrected. Figure 6b shows a presurgical topographical image of a bow tie keratoconus with a high central astigmatism, in which two flat-based segments of 150° arch and 6 mm diameter (represented at the center, below) are implanted. To the right, a postsurgical topographical image can be seen, where the astigmatism was corrected even though the cornea kept its prolaticity.

In conclusion, we can state that:

- Conical segments with 150° arch do not generate astigmatisms while maintaining corneal prolaticity and decreasing K values, whereas with 120°, the effect is to generate (or correct) small astigmatisms (up to 2.5 D).
- Flat segments with 150° arch: generate large astigmatisms in spherical corneas or can generate spherical effects on previous ectatic corneas.

All the effects of the segments can be summarized as follows:

- Diameter of the implants (ICRS): smaller diameter – greater effect; greater diameter –smaller effect (by Blastakya law representing an inverse relationship).
- Thickness of the implants (ICRS): less thickness – less effect; greater thickness – greater effect (by the other Blastakya law representing a direct relationship).
- Previous corneal K values where we implement ICRS: lower K values – less effect; higher K values –greater effect (direct relationship).

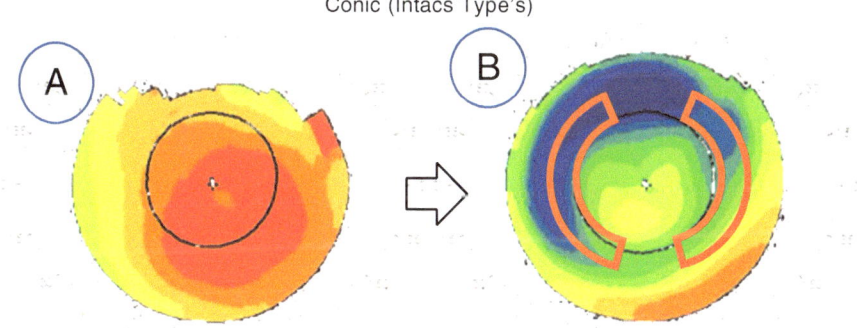

Cónic (Intacs Type's)

A

B

Fig. 5 (**a**) Presurgical spherical topography. (**b**) Post-op conic type's ICRS

Flattenet (Ferrara type's)

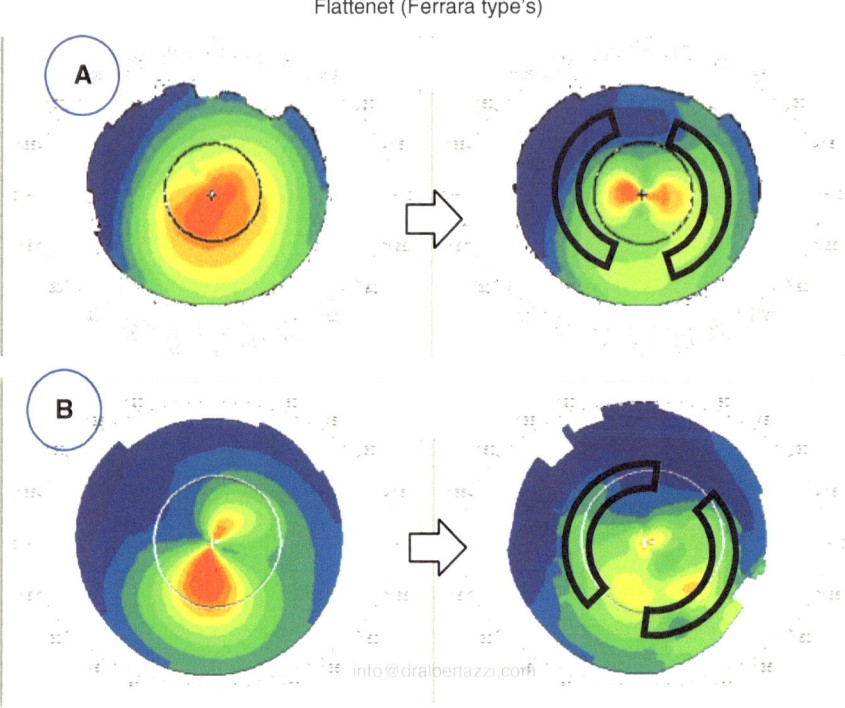

Fig. 6 (a) Left: presurgical spherical topography; right: Postop Ferrara type's ICRS. (b) Left: presurgical astigmatic topography; right: postop Ferrara type's ICRS

– Pachymetry where to implant ICRS: lower pachymetry – higher effect; higher pachymetry –lower effect (inverse relationship). This is as such if the ICRS is always at a depth of approximately 75% of the pachymetry.
– Implant depth: implants placed more superficially (50% stroma) will have more effect and will have more apical distal keratitis than those ICRS placed with more than 75% of depth.

ICRS rigidity and modification of the corneal structural behavior once implanted:

The stroma is stiff where the implant is and tension vectors are released at their ends. The conical profiles will release less tension, because their inclination is parallel to the cornea. Flat profiles will release much more tension, because their design opposes the corneal architecture and the 90–120° arch tension dissipates in a similar portion to that of the fabric, whereas those of 140–160° the dissipation of the effect is acquired at a lower percentage, where the most punctual effect occurs in the area. The large arches block this effect, evenly decreasing all corneal diopter values.

Once surpassing the 180° arch, a block of the release of the tension vectors at their ends and the whole pattern evenly lower the keratometric values, maintaining their topographic characteristics, though slightly smaller and more centered.

All arches maintain corneal prolaticity, even when used on hyperprolate corneas such as keratoconus.

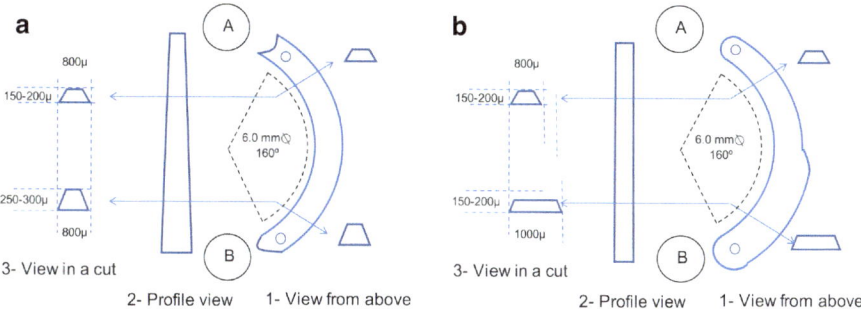

Fig. 7 Diagram of the asymmetric segments that were launched onto the market by Mediphacos at the end of 2015. The following can be observed: (1) overview: the segment has the same external and internal measurements, but different height, with two ends: A is the proximal end which is thinner and B is the distal end which is thicker. (2) Profile view: a gradual increase in volume from the height can be observed. (3) View of a cut: the real heights are shown, the segment which has 150 microns above and 250 microns below and the one which has 200 microns above and 300 microns below. The diameter is 6 mm and the base is about 800 microns.

Asymmetric Segments

These types of segments were described many years ago, but because of technical limitations, they were not successful on the market. These reached the market in 2015 in two versions: Mediphacos® – same base but increases the thickness and modifies the extremities as shown in Fig. 7a; Intraseg® – increases the distal base maintaining the thickness as shown in Fig. 7b.

The initial result of this design is good, even very good, but the appearance of the late apical chronic keratitis that can develop as a complication will be mentioned at the end of the chapter.

Corneal Ectasia: Classification Based on Their Origin and Structural Behavior

Ectasia After a Refractive Surgery (LASIK) (Fig. 8 – Left)

This is a very special kind of ectasia, with specific patterns and characteristics of having pathological values of corneal hysteresis; the tissue was considered normal and surgery was performed to achieve emmetropia; the aftermath had a sudden evolutionary and progressive pathology. All these characteristics give the impression of a surgical failure. This type of pathology represents a different behavior and includes a different treatment procedure from primary ectasias, since it doesn't share its structural functioning, nor its origin or its patterns, let alone its chronologic evolution.

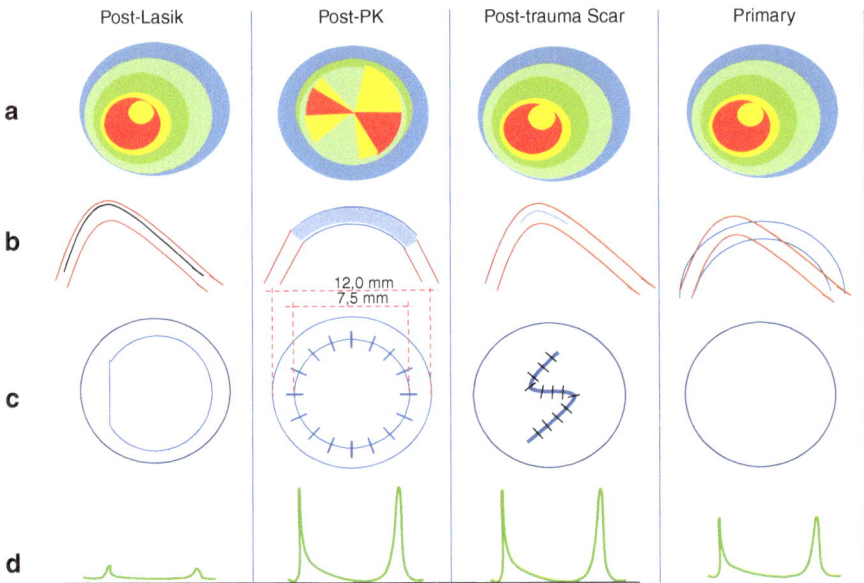

Fig. 8 Corneal ectasias: classification by their origin

Asymmetries Post Penetrating Keratoplasty (PK)

The circular scar of ± 7.5 mm, achieved from the corneal graft, functions as a structural neo-limbo, fluctuating until stability is reached (Fig. 8, center left).

These features create very special conditions (Fig. 8, center left) as they have the following:

1. Topographic patterns that have high asymmetry(Fig. 8a, center left)
2. The corneal scar is visible in full stroma (Fig. 8b, center left)
3. The BMC clearly shows the original high corneal button pachymetries, a corneal ring scar (Fig. 8c, center left)
4. Hysteresis is high for all these structural changes (Fig. 8d, center left)

All these characteristics cause loss in predictability with the intracorneal segments designed for ectasias. We need special designs of segments to attend this case.

Ectasia or Post-corneal Wounds (Fig. 8, Center Right)

The behavior of the labels sectioned traumatically makes the tissue evolve into a scar, unequal to others, since it depends on the architecture of the wound itself, which far from joining them, adheres them with fibrin, thus making the structural behavior also different:

1. Topographic patterns can reshape primary patterns (Fig. 8a, center right)
2. The corneal scar is visible in full stroma (Fig. 8b, center right)
3. The BMC clearly sees the origin (Fig. 8c, center right)
4. Hysteresis is high for all these structural changes (Fig. 8d, center right)

Primary Ectasia (Fig. 8, Right)

Although only one gene that can produce primary ectasias has been identified, the origin is still unknown, even though they are frequently familiar, congenital, hereditary, and bilateral with an asymmetric compromise.

The incidence described is that of 1:2000 inhabitants, with different characteristics within said population. For example, in the clinic where I work (Centro de Ojos Quilmes, Argentina), we are 84 workers and there are 2 patients with keratoconus, which means that in the universe of the clinic, the incidence is 2:84 much more than any other report.

The initial appearance is usually during the adolescence years, during which it has a faster progression, and must be treated with celerity when evolution of ectasia is found. In adulthood, the evolution is not so progressive, unless the cornea is subject of chronic aggressions due to improper use of contact lenses with defective adaptations, keratitis, and repetitive corneal ulcers. These are the main features:

1. They present defined stages and patterns, which are repeated in the population, suffering small alterations between them (Fig. 8a, right).
2. This is a deformation on a cornea that was normal (Fig. 8b, right).
3. Unless Vogt stretch marks are observed, they do not have BMC signs (Fig. 8c, right).
4. Alterations in hysteresis with subnormal values (Fig. 8d, right).

Patterns of Primary Ectasia

Patterns are a set of topography and tomography signs with which we classify ectasias. We can divide ectasias into paracentral or asymmetric and central or symmetric (Fig. 9).

When discussing *stages*, we refer to the degree of development of each of them (Fig. 10). The stages were described by Amsler-Krumeich [5] who developed a practical classification that contained very useful clinical, keratometric, and biomicroscopic data to quickly know the structural involvement of the cornea. They described four well-differentiated stages.

It was José Alfonso [6, 7] who described the anatomy in a more rational way due to a retrospective study of his database. Thus, based on the existing categories described, it divides ectasias into paracentral and central, as we have been doing since 2000, but identifies patterns, thanks to associating topographies with topographical planes and coma axis. He studied and described the relationship of the following:

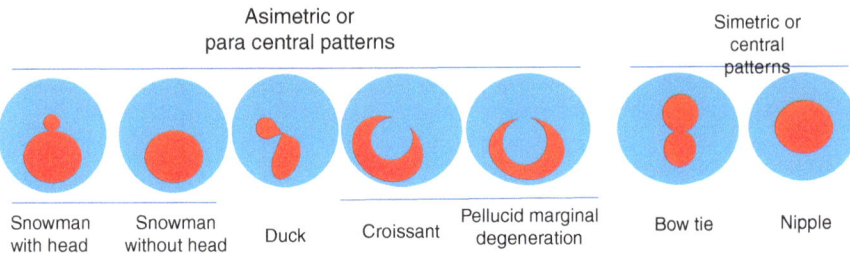

Fig. 9 Asymmetrical or paracentral patterns: (**a**) Snowman with and without head and (**b**) duck and (**c**) croissant. Symmetrical or central patterns: (**d**) bow tie and (**e**) nipple [4]

Fig. 10 This development is vital to get a quick idea of the structural behavior of the cornea [5]

1	Eccentric steepening,Myopia Induced astigmatism, or both ⟨5.00 D Mean central reading ⟨48 D
2	Myopia, induced astigmatism, or both from 5.00 to 8.00 D Mean central reading ⟨53 D Absence of scarring. Paquimetry ⟩ 400µ
3	Myopia, induced astigmatism, or both from 8.00 to 10.00 D Mean central reading ⟩ 53 D Absence of scarring. Paquimetry 300 - 400µ
4	Refraction not measurable Mean central reading ⟩ 55 D Central corneal scarring Paquimetry ⟨200 µ

- Visual axis and the thinner pachymetric point
- The deviation of the comatic axis in relation to the topographic axis

The association of the thinner pachymetric point has, in my opinion, better association than the comatic axes which can be confusing.

In the following chart, we will associate the stages with the topographic patterns plus in a series of 273 eyes operated from ICRS consecutively between 8/2016 and 8/2017. In Fig. 11, different stages of the sample are plotted.

Stages of Primary Ectasia

Stage 1
Stage 1 values up to 47D (±2D) Pachymetry of 470 µ (±30 µ) (where pachymetries are subnormal as well as keratometric values). This stage is found in a low percentage and usually corresponds to the opposite eye for which the patient consults.

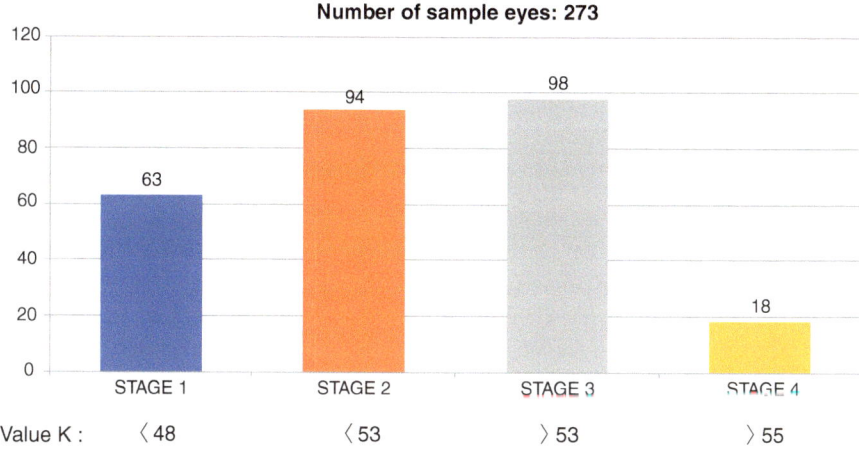

Fig. 11 Different stages of the sample

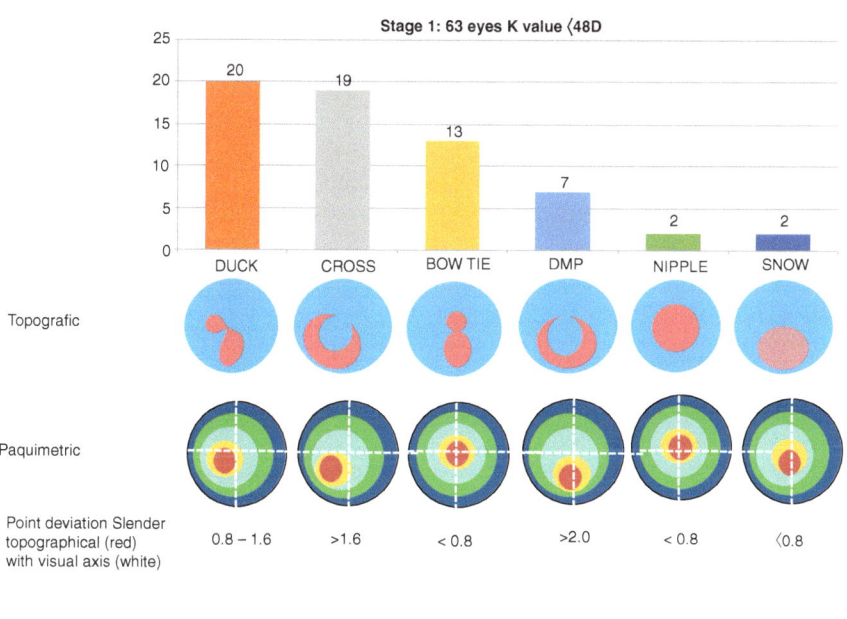

Fig. 12 Stage 1: Frequencies, pattern-type schemes, topographic images, and topographic planes, with the thinnest point and its deviation from the visual axis in millimeters

The thinnest areas of the pachymetry are indicated in red (Fig. 12) and below them the distances in millimeters that separate it from the visual axis. Perhaps the theory of sphere caps [8] can explain why a small optic area has more effect in producing an ectasia rather than a wide one.

Duck This pattern resembles a duck because one end is smaller than the other. It is considered asymmetrical and has other characteristics such as low and medium astigmatism that never exceed six [9] diopters and many of them are refracted with crossed cylinders. It has a high incidence and together with the croissant, are the two most frequent in all the initial stages.

Croissant This pattern resembles a crab claw, because the ends, unlike the afore-mentioned duck pattern, are symmetrical, perhaps because the thinnest pachymetric point is further away from the visual axis, causing more symmetry to its topographic presentation. The characteristic clinical signs are astigmatisms that are a little bit higher than those of the duck, are more symmetric, and the VA is usually better corrected than the duck patterns.

Bow Tie Here the thinnest point usually coincides with the visual axis, or is very close to it, which gives certain characteristics of its own, such as a very wide range in the astigmatic amount, from very high to medium to low.

They are usually symmetrical, with small asymmetries, but are always in favor of the rule, that is to say that the axis with the highest keratometric value is at 90°. When this vertical axis is slightly tilted, they become similar to ducks.

Pellucid Marginal Degeneration In this pattern, although confused with the croissant, pachymetric thinning is more peripherally located, with higher hypermetropic values, and its stromal refinements are usually extreme. Due to its location, it competes with a penetrating keratoplasty.

Nipple It is not common to find nipples in primary stages, but they are often diagnosed in the advanced stages of ectasias. The patterns have a high central keratometric values. They have diffused edges in topography presented with different diameters and are accompanied by a decrease in the central pachymetry.

Snowman with/without head These two patterns are grouped because they have similar characteristics: low astigmatism with topographic axes that differ almost 90° from the coma axes, making them very difficult to refract. Both patterns are infrequent.

Stage 2

Patients found in stage 2, shown in Fig. 13, may already have symptoms of visual decline, distortion, and daily fluctuations. The importance of topography-assisted refraction becomes more relevant, because it helps perform a correct surgical tactic. The Keratoconus Refraction Helper app provides a simple and correct guidance in this regard based on the premise of the preexisting emetropy prior to the ectasia, and any deformation of the corneal anterior face will lead to a distortion of its surface, modifying the K value.

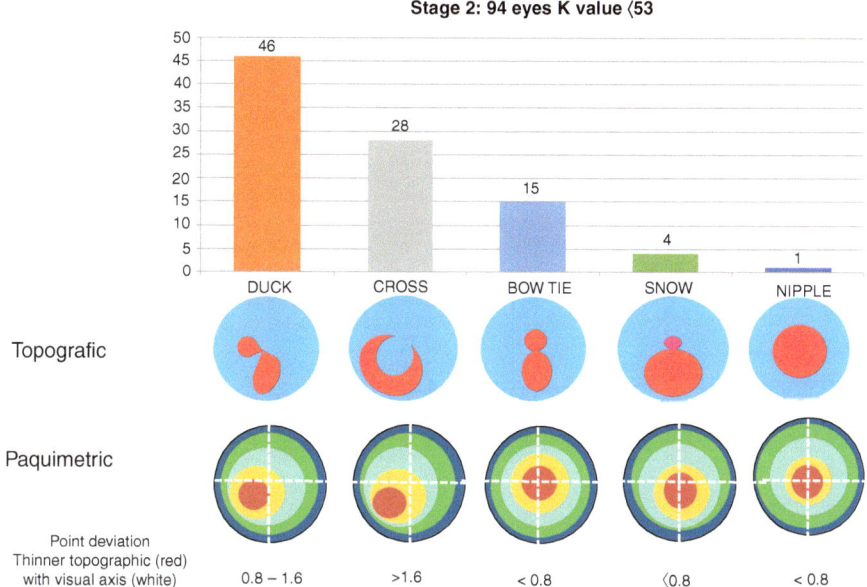

Fig. 13 Stage 2: frequencies, pattern-type schemes, topographic images, and topographic planes, with the thinnest point and its deviation from the visual axis in millimeters

If we give this K value a standard value of 43D, we can correct these patients: Everything that exceeds 43D will have to be corrected with myopic components and all lower keratometric values with hypermetropic components.

These patients no longer achieve a 10/10 BCVA (Best Corrected Visual Acuity) and rely on optical aids to improve their vision, and many of them begin to use contact lenses daily, since they give better vision quality.

Stage 3

At this stage, shown in Fig. 14, patients become very much aware of decreased vision, since it is usually associated with the appearance of fine vertical folds that cross the visual axis, called Vogt's striae, and pachymetric thinning areas are wider with respect to their previous locations.

The treatment here is tectonic rather than refractive.

Stage 4

In this stage, shown in Fig. 15, the corneal alteration is complete and widespread.

Treatment with ICRS will only be considered if there are no scars in the visual axis and if the patient has phobias to surgery or is very young. Such patients are not

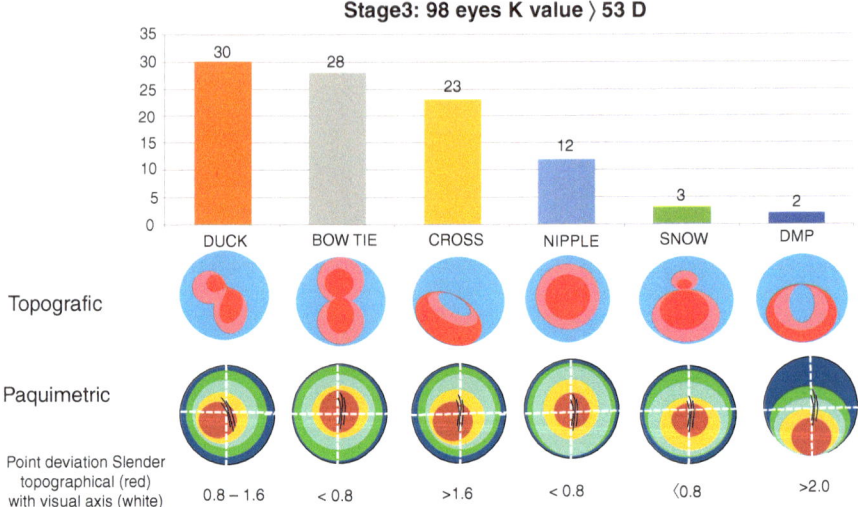

Fig. 14 Stage 3: frequencies, pattern-type schemes, topographic images, and topographic planes, with the thinnest point and its deviation from the visual axis in millimeters

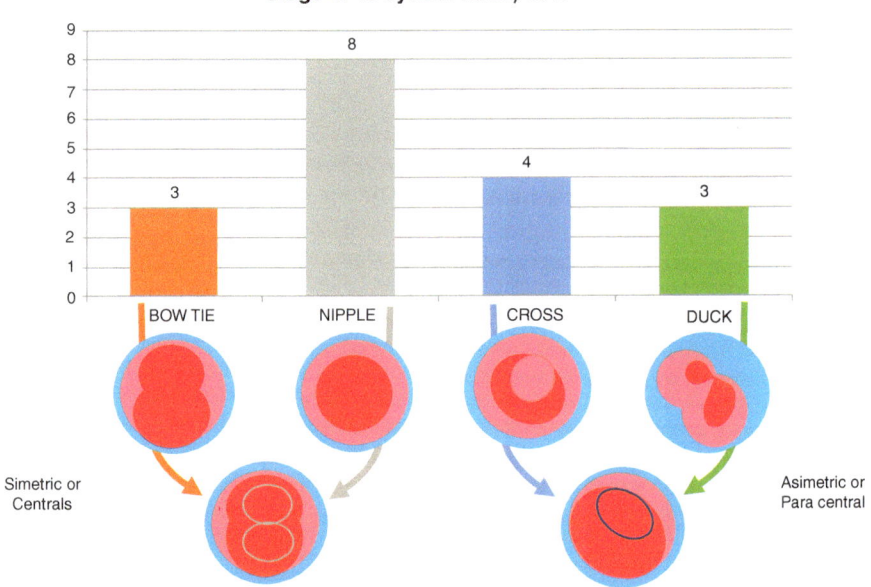

Fig. 15 Stage 4: frequencies, pattern-type schemes, topographic images, and their transformation into symmetrical patterns on the left and asymmetrical on the right

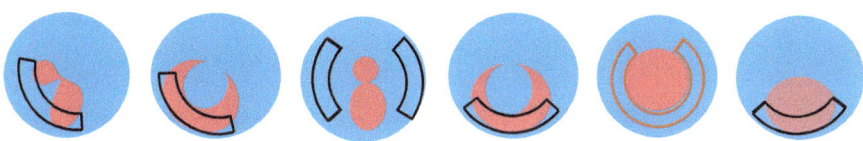

Fig. 16 Treatment scheme the most frequently found patterns of stage 1, in black flat profiles, in red, conical profiles

good candidates for ICRS and their vision will depend on the postsurgical adaptation of scleral support contact lenses.

ICRS Treatment in Stage 1

The indications of stage 1 are shown in Fig. 16. Segments here will have refractive objective [10, 11].

In the ducks, the astigmatisms are low, no more than 3 diopters are found, and usually only one inferior temporal segment is needed.

The croissants also show low astigmatisms in these stages and are very similar to the ducks.

If bow ties are low, either one or two symmetrical segments are placed with very little effect.

In the pellucid marginal degeneration, the treatment is similar to that of the croissants.

In the snowman without a head, a lower segment will be sufficient if the patient refracts with an astigmatism against the rule, which is usually low.

The indication to insert only one segment in these stages is because it is not good to hypercorrect as the corneal structure functions resemble a waterbed. If we place the segment on a meridian, then the contralateral hemi-cornea curvatures increase.

Postoperatively, they will be very close to emmetropia (curvature).

The characteristics of these stages are as follows:

- The patients see well and present low ametropias in which the refraction matches the topography patterns.
- The corneal structure still works, which means that many get very close to emmetropia with only one segment (asymmetric ectasias). They need little effect and the volume must be in accordance with the pachymetry.

ICRS Treatment in Stadium 2

Amsler-Krumeich stage II: values from D47 (±2D) to D52 (±2D). The percentage of patients who consult in this stage is already high. Almost 40% of the surgery has the purpose of altering the development of an ectasia, modifying some of its structure and strengthening the tissue that remains between the limbo and the implant.

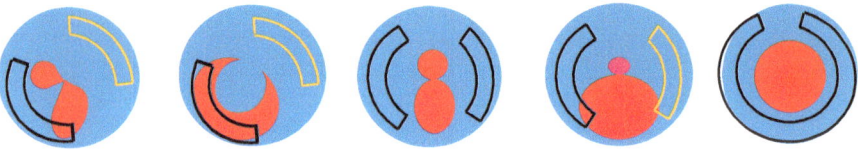

Fig. 17 Scheme for treating the most common primary ectasia patterns in stage 2

These are the most common indications, as shown in Fig. 17, where we modify some of its refraction without reaching 20/20 without correction postoperatively [10]. In the refractive aspect, there are low spherical remnants, due to the coupling effect resulting from the treatment of the astigmatic value.

Here we no longer have a snowman without head, and only a snowman with head will be present, though this is uncommon. It is possible to find different types of bow ties such as small, asymmetric, and inverted ones.

The characteristics of this stage are as follows:

- The patients have ametropia that reaches 0.6/0.8 with aerial correction.
- The refraction is in accordance with the topography patterns.
- The corneal structure does not work properly.

It is usually necessary to apply two segments to achieve more effect. This achieved effect has a post-surgical coupling that is presented as a residual spherical correction. They need more segment volume than in stage I.

Stage 3
The fundamental characteristics of these stages are the presence of Vogt's striae with a consequent decrease in visual acuity that cannot be corrected, so the indications will be tectonic.

These are palliative indications, shown in Fig. 18, where the implant only provides a paralimbar support of an unhealthy cornea in the patient who does not tolerate contact lenses and does not want to undergo a corneal graft [12].

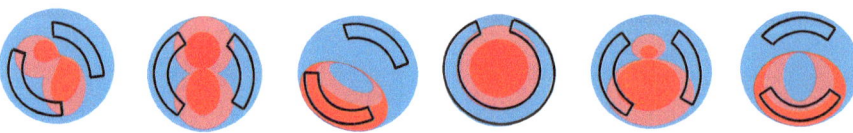

Fig. 18 Scheme for treating the most common primary ectasia patterns at stage 3

Simetric or
centrals

Asimetric or
para central

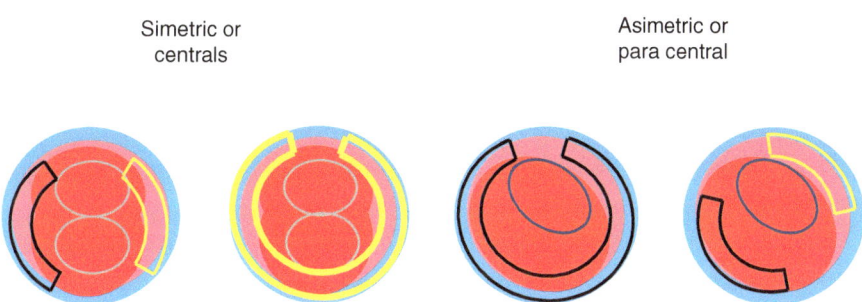

Fig. 19 Treatment of ectasias in stadium 4: We choose here to graph this stage with two patterns: central dominance (type A) or peripheral dominance (type B). Black segments illustrate flat type and yellow segments illustrate conical type

Stage 4

We choose here to graph this stage with two patterns: central predominance (type A) or a peripheral predominance (type B).

The treatment will be with medium (150–160°) or large (320°) arch segments, if possible conical or a combination of both, as shown in Fig. 19.

If flat segments are chosen, they should not be too high in thickness because of two reasons: (1) they do not have a lot of pachymetric thickness to support them and (2) they may produce a high astigmatism, where previously did not exist.

These stages are characterized by the following features:

- Larger pachymetric thinning.
- It's the rule to find Vogt's striae within the Descemet's membrane with a consequent decrease in visual acuity.
- They will never achieve 10/10 with correction but may be corrected partially with scleral lens.
- The effect sought here is only tectonic and not refractive.
- Tangential topographies tend to saturate the colors, making it impossible to find central patterns in this type of stage. For this reason, one should choose the axial ones.
- Within the axial topographies, I prefer the standardized scales that saturate less in order to find central patterns.
- Once these (patterns) are found, choose the axis where you will align the incision.
- Longer segments are used, usually matched at 150°.
- The purpose is to recover the surface and the corneal structure in order to be able to tolerate the adaptation of scleral lenses.
- It is very difficult to measure them because they have high myopic curvature.

Chronic Apical Distal and Late Keratitis (CADLK)

These appear at the distal end of the flat segments, and due to their mechanism of action, they always cause protrusion of their most curved edges (Figs. 20 and 21), which are the same as the lower ones, and more so when they are thicker. Figure 8 shows a case of CADLK, where thickness is only 150° microns.

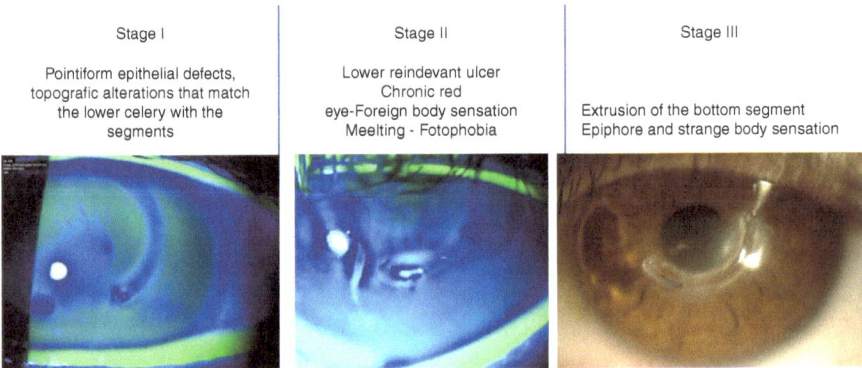

Fig. 20 Different stages of chronic apical and distal keratitis for ICRS (Albertazzi)

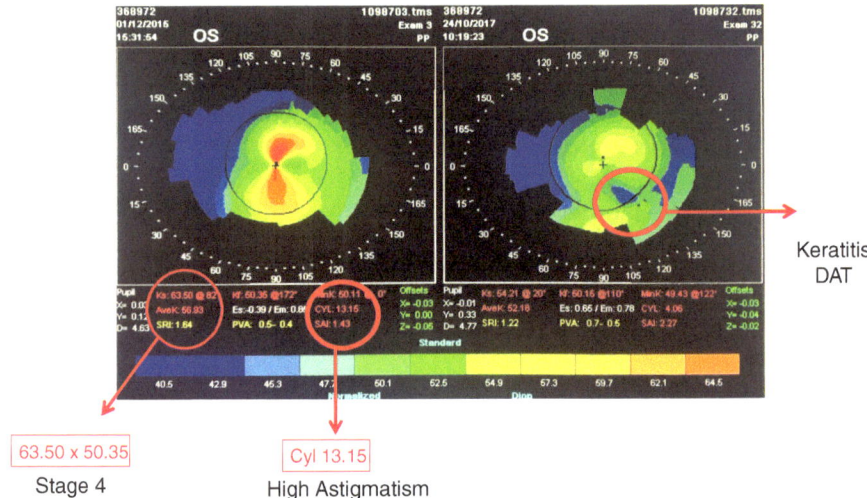

Fig. 21 Shows the pre- and post-surgical topography of a patient with CADLK: 1 – high keratometric values (63), 2 – high astigmatism (13 Dioptries), 3 – good post-surgical result but in the distal end of the temporal segment, a CADLK sign is already observed topographically as observed in the areas of low *K* values

Bibliographic References

1. Intacs – Surgeon Training Manual-For the correction of myopia. Pag 20 MK-US-50024-01-TOC/Rev.
2. Patent Application Publication Albertazzi: Intracorneal Implant and Injector to treat corneal disorder US 2019/0159888A1. 2019.
3. Blavatskaia ED. Intralamellar Homoplasty for the purpose of relaxation of refraction of the eye. Oftalmol Zh. 1968;7:530–7.
4. De Rojas Silva V. Clasificacion del Queratocono. In: En Albertazzi R, editor. Queratocono: pautas para su diagnostico y tratamiento. Buenos Aires, Ediciones Cientificas Argentinas; 2010. p. 33–97.
5. Krumeich JH, et al. Live-epikeratophakia for keratoconus. J Cataract Refract Surg. 1998;24:456–63.
6. Alfonso J, et al. Intrastromal corneal ring implantation in paracentral keratoconus with coincident topographic and coma axis. J Cataract Refract Surg. 2012;38:1576–82.
7. Fernandez-Vega Cueto L, Lisa C, Poo-Lopez A, et al. Intrastromal corneal ring segment implantation in 409 paracentral keratoconic eyes. Cornea. 2016;35:1421–6.
8. Carriazo C, Cosentino MJ. A novel corneal remodeling technique for the management of keratoconus. J Refract Surg. 2017;33(12):854–7.
9. Albertazzi Roberto G. Anatomia de un aectasia-World Keratoconus Society Meeting 14–17 mayo 2014.
10. Patent Application Publication Albertazzi: Methods and apparatus for treating keratoconus: US 9,931,199 B2. 2018.
11. Fahd DC, Alameddine RM, Nasser M, Awwad ST. Refractive and topographic effects of single-segment intrastromal corneal ring segments in eyes with moderate to severe keratoconus and inferior cones. J Cataract Refract Surg. 2015;41:1434–40.
12. Colin J, et al. Correcting keratoconus with intracorneal rings. J Cataract Refract Surg. 2000;26(8):1117–22.

Phakic Intraocular Lens in Keratoconus

Alaa Eldanasoury, Sherif Tolees, and Harkaran S. Bains

Keratoconus (KC) is a bilateral chronic, asymmetric, progressive disease that compromises the structural integrity of the collagen matrix in the corneal stoma [1, 2]. The prevalence of keratoconus varies widely based on geographic location. For example, the prevalence is 265 cases per 100,000 in the Netherlands and 4000 cases per 1000,000 in Iran [3, 4]. In Jordan, 5% of blindness among adults is due keratoconus [5]. The prevalence of keratoconus is much higher in the Middle East than in other regions due to genetic and environmental risk factors, such as consanguinity, sun exposure (ultraviolet exposure), eye rubbing, and nicotine use [6, 7].

Patients with keratoconus tend to self-select and present for refractive surgery screening looking to improve their poor visual acuity [8]. However, keratoconus is a contraindication for excimer laser refractive surgery. The hallmark of keratoconus is the development of a localized cone-shaped ectasia with thinning of the stroma in the area of the cone. These corneal changes initially manifest as corneal topographic changes. Early keratoconus can be detected with corneal topography of the anterior corneal surface before other clinical signs appear (Fig. 1) [8–10]. The topographic changes include [8, 10] a local area of abnormal steepening often located inferiorly and more advanced topographic changes in one eye compared to the fellow eye with

Electronic Supplementary Material The online version of this chapter (https://doi.org/10.1007/978-3-030-66143-4_7) contains supplementary material, which is available to authorized users.

A. Eldanasoury · S. Tolees (✉)
Department of Ophthalmology, Magrabi Hospital, Jeddah, Saudi Arabia
e-mail: Sherif.Tolees@magrabi.com.sa

H. S. Bains
Sight By Design, Edmonton, AB, Canada

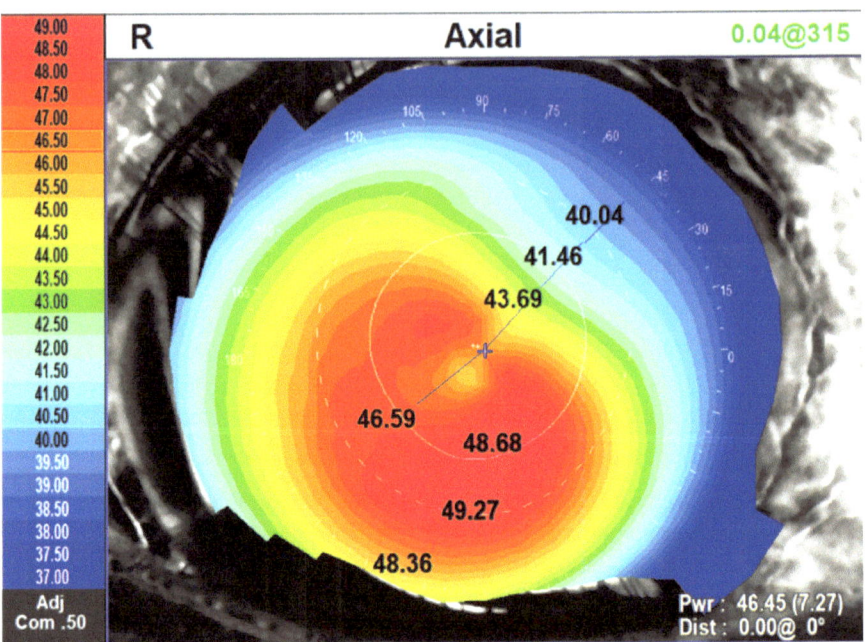

Fig. 1 Axial topography map of early keratoconus (OPD Scan III, NIDEK Co. Ltd.)

nonsuperimposable mirror-image symmetry but similar patterns. This localized conical shape induces lower-order refractive error such as myopia, high regular and irregular astigmatism, and other higher-order aberrations (HOAs) resulting in a concurrent degradation of visual quality [1, 2, 11]. The course of the disease varies from slight irregular astigmatism to severe visual impairment due the progression of the cone and stromal scarring [4]. Keratoconus can be classified based on the Amsler-Krumeich criteria into four stages based on severity [12, 13].

Generally, visual rehabilitation for keratoconic corneas requires addressing three concerns: halting the progressive ectasia, improving corneal shape, and minimizing residual refractive error. Treatment modalities vary based on the stages of keratoconus. Spectacles, soft lenses, soft toric, or custom soft toric contact lenses may be used for patients with early KC who have myopia, regular astigmatism, and mildly irregular astigmatism. However, as the disease progresses resulting in significant irregular astigmatism and anisometropia, satisfactory vision can be achieved with rigid gas-permeable (RGP) lenses or various specialized lenses, such as hybrid, piggyback, or scleral lenses [14]. For advanced cases that cannot be corrected with RGP or specialty lenses and contact lens-intolerant cases, surgical treatment is warranted. Surgical options included penetrating keratoplasty (PKP) or deep anterior lamellar keratoplasty (DALK) [14].

If the disease is progressive with acceptable corrected visual acuity, corneal collagen cross-linking (CXL) using riboflavin and UV light can effectively halt the progression [15]. However the residual refractive error requires correction with contact lenses, intracorneal ring segments, or spectacles.

The hallmarks of progressive keratoconus include one or more of the following occurring within a year: an increase in astigmatism of 1.0 D or greater, significant change in the orientation of the refractive axes, an increase of 1.0 D or greater in the steepest corneal meridian, and a decrease of at least 25 μm in corneal thickness [1, 2].

In patients with stable keratoconus, the associated refractive error can be corrected with various modalities including intracorneal ring segments, contact lenses, and phakic intraocular lenses (pIOLs) [14, 16, 17]. Phakic IOLs can correct high refractive error and offer the advantages of maintaining accommodation and a reversible procedure. Currently, there are three types of pIOLs: angle-supported anterior chamber pIOLs, iris-claw anterior chamber pIOLs, and collamer posterior chamber (PC) pIOLs [18–20].

Phakic Intraocular Lenses

The US Food and Drug Administration (FDA) approved the Verisyse iris-claw pIOL (Abbott Laboratories Inc., Abbott Park, IL, USA) and Visian collamer PC pIOL (STAAR Surgical Co, Monrovia, CA, USA). Both of these pIOLs are approved for patients with high myopia and low astigmatism (<2.5 D). Toric pIOLs are not currently FDA approved. In Europe, the Artisan pIOL (Ophtec BV, the Netherlands) and newer models of various pIOLs including toric pIOLs have received the CE mark. All angle-supported phakic lenses have been withdrawn from the market due to complications mainly related to endothelial loss.

The iris-fixated pIOL for the correction of myopia was introduced by Worst and Fechner in 1986 as a rigid single-piece Polymethyl methacrylate (PMMA) model with a 5.0 or 6.0 mm optic [18–20]. These phakic lenses are based on the principle of iris fixation. This method of intraocular fixation does not restrict constriction and dilation of the pupil and ensures stable fixation to the iris due to the two diametrically opposed haptics allowing lens centration over the pupil. Over time the lens design was modified to a convex-concave Artisan myopia lens. The new design decreased the potential for complications, improved the optical performance, and facilitated the surgical implantation technique. In 2005 and 2009, the Artiflex myopia lens and Artiflex toric lens were introduced into the market, respectively. The foldable design with a silicone optic and PMMA haptics facilitates implantation through a 3.2 mm incision. Complications of iris-fixated pIOLs include recurrent intraocular inflammation, enhanced iris dispersion with posterior synechiae, and lenticular glistering [17, 18].

Currently, two posterior chamber phakic IOLs are available, the implantable collamer lens (ICL) (Staar Surgical Co.) and the phakic refractive lens (PRL) (Carl Zeiss Meditec). The ICL is currently the most widely used posterior chamber phakic IOL as the PRL is rapidly falling out of favor over the last few years due to a variety of complications.

The ICL is comprised of collamer that is a highly biocompatible hydrophilic porcine collagen/hydroxyethyl methacrylate copolymer, with an ultraviolet-absorbing chromophore. The Visian ICL V4 incorporates an additional vault compared to the previous model for greater clearance between the posterior surface of the ICL and the anterior surface of the crystalline lens. The Visian ICL V4 can correct spherical refractive error ranging from −18 to +10 D, and the Visian toric ICL can correct cylinder up to 6.0 D.

In May 2017, the EVO+ Visian ICL with aspheric optic received CE mark. This version (V5) of the lens has an expanded optical zone (6.1 mm optic) that allows implantation in patients with larger pupils (to reduce diffraction effect, such as halos). The V4c and V5 models have a central hole with a diameter of 0.36 mm which circumvents the need for a peripheral iridotomy and increases aqueous humor perfusion, thereby reducing the risk of secondary cataract formation [21].

Criteria for Phakic Intraocular Lens Implantation in Keratoconus Patients

The criteria for keratoconus patients who are candidates for pIOL implantation include age between 20 and 45 years, contact lens intolerance, normal systemic history, normal physical examination, absence of any history or physical signs of ocular disease other than keratoconus and myopia, a stable refraction for at least 12 months, corrected distance visual acuity (CDVA) of 0.3 (20/60) or better in the eye to be treated (with the lowest sphere and cylinder values that give the corrected distance visual acuity), stable spectacle power for at least 1 year defined as a change in power less than 0.50 D MRSE, stable corneal topography, a clear central cornea, a normal anterior segment with an anterior chamber depth of at least 3.00 mm, and a normal intraocular pressure.

Stable refraction is defined as a change of 0.50 D or less in manifest refractive spherical equivalent (MRSE) yearly. Patient satisfaction with spectacle power can be verified by a 2-week trial of the prescription. If the patient is satisfied with the vision, the postoperative visual performance is expected to be satisfactory. Stable corneal topography can be verified by differential topography (Fig. 2). Anterior chamber depth can be measured using IOL Master (Carl Zeiss, Jena, Germany), a Scheimpflug anterior segment imaging (e.g., Pentacam), or anterior segment OCT (Fig. 3).

Combined Placido and OCT technology such as the MS-39 (CSO, Firenze, Italy) provides important data such as HVID (horizontal visible iris diameter), the measurement of the horizontal limbus diameter (in mm), and HACD (horizontal anterior chamber diameter), the measurement of the distance between the vertices of the iridocorneal angles. These diameters are derived from the Placido image. Crystalline lens rise is the difference between the position of the crystalline lens and the iridocorneal plane, i.e., the best-fit plane "passing" through the vertices of the

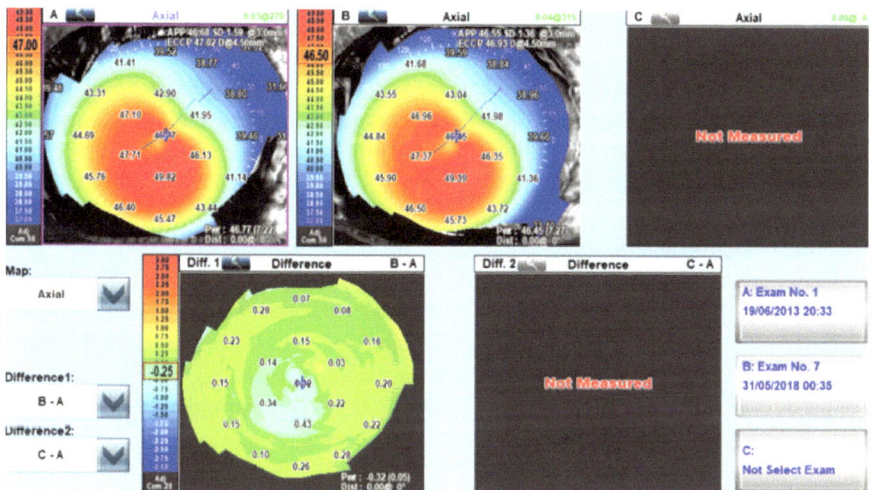

Fig. 2 Differential map showing stable keratoconus for 5-year SP cross-linking (OPD Scan III, NIDEK Co. Ltd.)

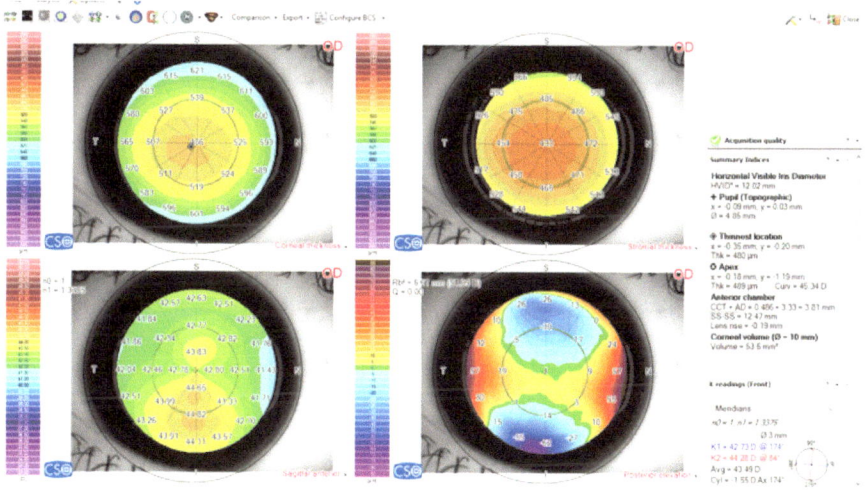

Fig. 3 MS-39 map showing the summary indices of the anterior chamber (Zeus MS-39, CSO)

iridocorneal angles. A negative value means that the crystalline lens is above the iridocorneal plane.

Contraindications for pIOL implantation in keratoconics include progressive keratoconus, unstable corneas, patients less than 20 years old, and highly aberrated eyes (total higher-order aberrations >3 μm) with poor CDVA of less than 0.5 LogMAR (20/60).

Phakic Intraocular Lens Power Calculation

As we routinely implant the ICL for patients with stable keratoconus, we will describe the power calculation of this lens. ICL power is calculated using the software provided by the manufacturer targeting emmetropia. The stable subjective refraction, as described above, is used to calculate ICL power. The appropriate size of the ICL is determined based on manual measurement of horizontal white-to-white distance with a caliper, and the anterior chamber depth is measured with the Pentacam.

In cases of advanced anterior corneal protrusion, a minor clinical adjustment of anterior chamber depth is performed by subtracting no more than 0.2 mm. Previous studies have documented how to optimize the final central vault of the ICL in eyes with keratoconus and myopia to ensure implantation of an adequately sized lens (Fig. 4) [22]. An oversized pIOL (e.g., lens is too long) can push the iris forward, decreasing angle clearance. An undersized pIOL (e.g., lens is too short) can result in the absence of vault (pIOL-crystalline lens touch), increasing the risk for early anterior subcapsular cataract. The length of the pIOL is selected based on the white-to-white (WTW) distance or the sulcus-to-sulcus (STS) distance using the manufacturer's protocol. A study of the final central vault distance at 3 months postoperatively or longer indicated that the WTW and STS methods both provided adequate final central vault in keratoconic eyes with myopia [22].

Currently Anterior segment optical coherence tomography (AS-OCT) is a useful tool for ICL size determination because it calculates the anterior segment parameters using automated analysis and the reproducibility is high. The NK formula has been developed for higher accuracy for predicting safe vault size than the STAAR nomogram. It depends on two main parameters, the distance between scleral spurs (anterior chamber width (ACW)) and crystalline lens rise (CLR) (Fig. 3) [23].

Manufactures of toric pIOLs include a guide documenting the required amount and direction of rotation from the horizontal axis to achieve the cylinder correction. Power calculation for iris-claw pIOLs is calculated with the Van der Heijde formula and includes patient refraction, keratometry, and adjusted ultrasound anterior

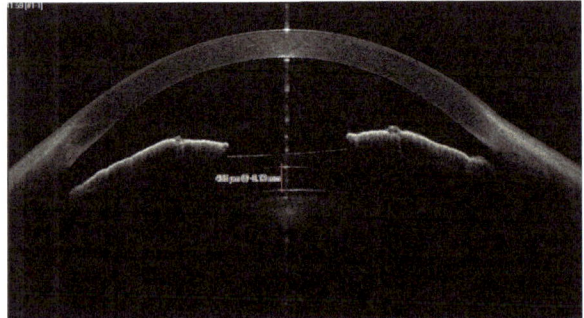

Fig. 4 Anterior segment optical coherence tomography showing measurement of implantable collamer lens vault (455 microns) (Zeus MS-39, CSO)

chamber depth (ACD). The manufacturer provides nomograms or software to calculate the pIOL power based on this formula. The iris-claw PIOL has an overall
fixed diameter of 8.5 mm.

Implantable Collamer Lens for Keratoconus

Our experience with ICLs spans over a decade. Here we present our surgical technique and current outcomes in patients with keratoconus.

Surgery (Video 1)

Thirty minutes prior to surgery, the pupil is dilated with instillation of cyclopento-
late and phenylephrine drops. In patients undergoing toric ICL (TICL) implantation, the surgeon marks the horizontal axis with the patient sitting upright to
control for cyclotorsion when the patient is supine. All patients undergo surgery
with topical anesthesia and oral sedation. The eye is prepared in a sterile fashion
and draped, and after instillation of topical anesthetic, a lid speculum is placed for
maximum globe exposure. For patients receiving a TICL, a Mendez ring is used
for intraoperative measurement of rotation from the horizontal axis. Recently, we
have used a digital alignment (without any ink marks) using eye images captured
by IOL Master (Carl Zeiss Meditec AG, Jena, Germany). The information, including corneal astigmatism data, is transferred to the Callisto eye system (Carl Zeiss
Meditec AG, Jena, Germany). This system superimposes templates of the lens
target axis over the eye in the eyepiece and heads-up display in the Zeiss microscope matching the reference image of the patient's eye and tracks the eye in real
time. After filling the cartridge with viscoelastic material, the lens is carefully
removed from the bottle with non-toothed forceps and placed on a foam tip to
avoid any damage. The footplate marks on the leading right and trailing left haptic
indicate that the correct convex side of the ICL is facing up. The ICL is placed in
the cartridge bay with a convex configuration, so that the long axis of the ICL is
positioned in the groove under each side rail of the cartridge. Coaxial forceps are
used to slowly pull the ICL into the barrel until the leading edge is adjacent to the
end of the cartridge. The cartridge is placed into the front of the injector and snap-
locked in place. The plunger is advanced until the foam tip is in contact with the
edge of the lens. The final ICL position should be within 2 mm of the end of the
cartridge.

A 3.0 mm clear corneal incision is performed in the horizontal temporal meridian, and the anterior chamber was filled with sodium hyaluronate 1%. A loaded ICL
is inserted into the posterior chamber through the incision using the injector cartridge. The cartridge is inserted bevel-down, and the lens is carefully injected in the

anterior chamber. Twisting the bevel right or left can be helpful in controlling lens unfolding and to maintain the correct lens orientation. The temporal subincisional footplates are manipulated by a blunt manipulator and positioned under the iris in the sulcus. Subsequently a 1 mm side port size is created 90° from the temporal incision to enable easier implantation of the leading footplates in the sulcus.

After the ICL is gently positioned in the sulcus with the axis properly aligned, a thorough irrigation with balanced salt solution is used to remove the remaining viscoelastic material from the anterior chamber, and a topical miotic is instilled. A vitrectomy cutter is used to create a surgical iridectomy after pupil constriction is achieved. As the ICL model V4C onward contains a central hole, this step is seldomly performed except for hyperopic eyes. Subsequently, an intracameral injection of antibiotic is delivered followed by stromal hydration for sealing the corneal wounds.

Care should be taken while creating the incision as the thin cornea in keratoconics may result in early entry into the anterior chamber with a short tunnel created by the main wound. This short tunnel may induce frequent iris prolapse during the manipulation and may leak at the end of the surgery. An interrupted suture may be required if stromal hydration does not seal the incision.

Bilateral surgical procedures must be handled as two separate procedures with separate batch numbers for disposables and on different tables.

Outcomes

We evaluated the outcomes of implantation of posterior chamber pIOL (ICL/TICL) for the correction of refractive error in 50 eyes with stable keratoconus.

Postoperative follow-up for 3 years or longer is presented here.

The mean age of all patients was 29 years (range 20–43 years). Fifty-four percent (27/50) of patients were female. Fifty percent (25/50) of right eyes and 50% (25/50) of left eyes underwent ICL implantation. Table 1 presents the distribution of TICL or ICL implantation as a primary or secondary procedure. At 1 year postoperatively,

Table 1 Distribution of the type of implantable collamer lens in patients with stable keratoconus as a primary or secondary procedure

	ICL (eyes)	TICL (eyes)	Total (eyes)
Stable KC	20	13	33
SP CXL	6	10	16
SP ICRS	0	1	1
Total	26	24	50

KC denotes keratoconus, *SP* denotes status post, *CXL* denotes corneal cross-linking, *ICL* denotes implantable collamer lens, *TICL* denotes toric ICL, *ICRS* denotes intracorneal ring segment

50 eyes (follow-up rate 100%) were available for follow-up. At 3 years postoperatively, 27 eyes (follow-up rate 54%) were available for follow-up. Table 2 presents the mean preoperative and postoperative refractive error. At 1 year postoperatively, the majority of eyes (94%) were within 1.00 D of the intended correction (Fig. 5). Stability is presented in Fig. 6. At 1 year postoperatively, 52% of the eyes gained one or more lines of CDVA, and 2% of the eyes lost CDVA (Fig. 7). Preoperative CDVA compared to postoperative uncorrected distance visual acuity (UDVA) is presented in Fig. 8.

Mean endothelial cell count was 2665.14 ± 200.73 cells/mm^2 (range 2333–3165 cells/mm^2) preoperatively and 2627 ± 297.65 cells/mm^2 (range 2069–3123 cells/mm^2) at 1 year postoperatively.

There were no intraoperative complications. Postoperatively, no eyes required explantation, and no cases of TICLs required repositioning (Video 2). At 3 years postoperatively, there were no postoperative complications, specifically, there were no cases of a decentered optic or pupillary block.

Table 2 Preoperative and postoperative refraction of patient with stable keratoconus who received an implantable collamer lens as a primary or secondary procedure

	Preoperative (n = 50 eyes)	1 year post-op (n = 50 eyes)	3 years post-op (n = 27 eyes)
SE (D)	−5.85 D ± 4.14 (range −16.75 to −1.00)	−0.21 D ± 0.60 (range −2.00 to 1.00)	−0.32 D ± 0.46 D (range −1.88 to 0.63)
Sphere (D)	−5.07 D ± 3.94 (range −16.00 to 0.00)	0.12 ± 0.60 (range −1.75 to 1.75)	−0.03 D ± 0.46 D (range −1.50 to 1.25)
Cylinder (D)	−1.56 D ± 1.45 (range −6.00 to 0.00)	−0.66 ± 0.55 (range −2.25 to 0.00)	−0.59 D ± 0.46 D (range −1.50 to 0.00)

SE denotes spherical equivalent

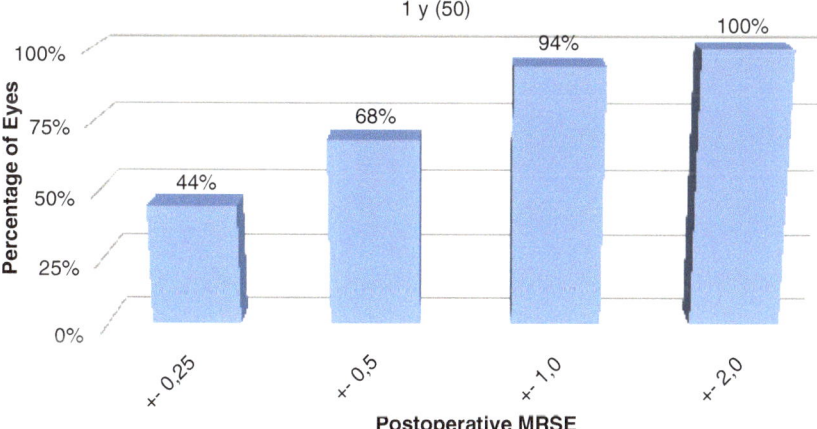

Fig. 5 Refractive outcomes at 1 year postoperatively of eyes with stable keratoconus that underwent implantable collamer lens implantation as a primary or secondary procedure

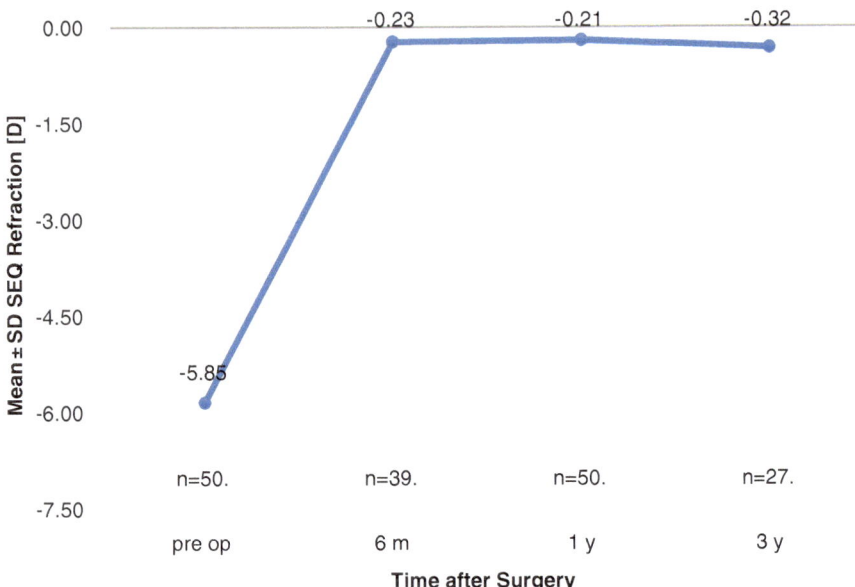

Fig. 6 Change in mean spherical equivalent over time of eyes with stable keratoconus that underwent implantable collamer lens implantation as a primary or secondary procedure. SEQ denotes manifest refractive spherical equivalent. Error bars indicate standard deviation

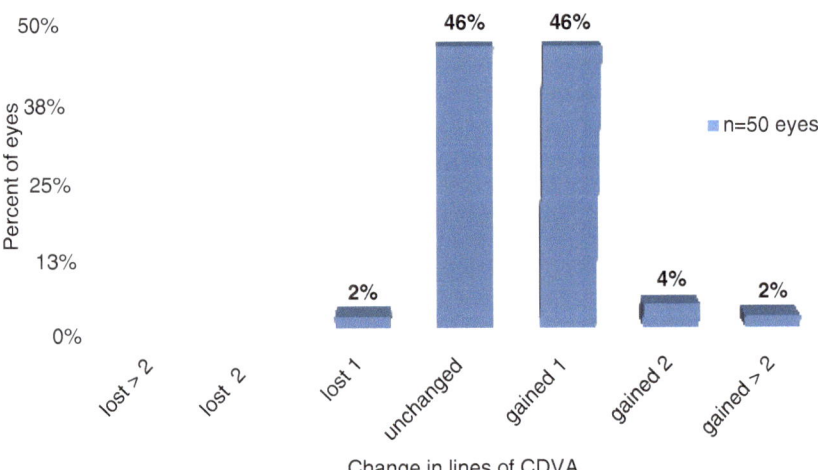

Fig. 7 Change in corrected distance visual acuity (CDVA) 1 year after of eyes with stable keratoconus that underwent implantable collamer lens implantation as a primary or secondary procedure. Gained >2 denotes greater than a 2-line gain of CDVA, gained 2 denotes a 2-line gain of CDVA, lost 1 indicates a 1-line loss of CDVA, lost 2 indicates a 2-line loss of CDVA, and lost >2 indicates greater than a 2-line loss of CDVA

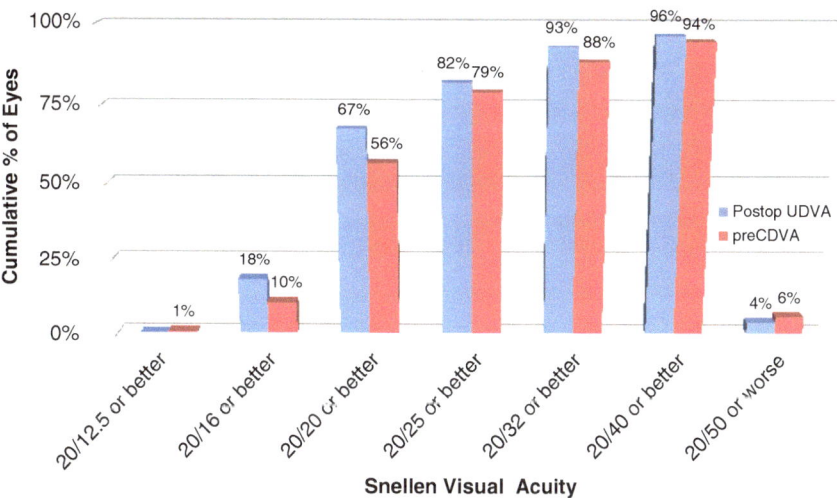

Fig. 8 Preoperative corrected distance visual acuity (CDVA) compared to postoperative uncorrected distance visual acuity (UDVA) in eyes with stable keratoconus that underwent implantable collamer lens implantation as a primary or secondary procedure

Summary

Phakic IOLs are a good option for treatment of ametropia associated with keratoconus and are a potential alternative to spectacles. However, pIOLs are also a treatment for ectasia. The use of pIOLs should be limited to patients with stable disease that must be documented on repeat visits using stringent screening criteria. Excimer laser surgery for stable keratoconus carries the risk of precipitating postoperative ectasia. Keratoconic eyes that have undergone corneal cross-linking have been treated with photorefractive keratectomy [24, 25]. However, the potential benefits of corneal cross-linking are reduced when the excimer laser ablates some of the cross-linked cornea. Furthermore, recent studies have reported postoperative complications of delayed epithelial healing and corneal haze in eyes that have undergone corneal cross-linking combined with photorefractive keratectomy [24].

Alfonso et al. (2008) [26] investigation of 25 eyes of ICL implantation for the correction of myopia associated with keratoconus reported a mean MRSE of 0.32 ± 0.55 D, 1 year postoperatively, which is somewhat different than our outcome of -0.21 ± 0.60 D postoperatively. A study of the ICL implantation in 30 eyes after corneal cross-linking for keratoconus reported 20/30 or better UDVA at 1 year postoperatively which is somewhat lower than our outcome of 93% (Fig. 8) [27]. The mean postoperative MRSE from our study are similar to Güell et al. (2012) $(-0.22$ D) and lower than Venter's (2009) outcomes (0.13 D) (Table 3) [28, 29].

The safety of pIOL implantation as primary or secondary procedure for stable keratoconus has been consistently demonstrated in numerous studies [26–32]. For

Table 3 Outcomes of studies evaluating primary or secondary phakic intraocular lens implantation for the treatment of refractive error associated with keratoconus

Study	# of eyes	Type of pIOL	1° or 2° procedure	Pre-op MRSE (D)	Post-op MRSE (D)	Loss of ≥2 lines CDVA	Post-op UDVA (LogMAR)	Post-op CDVA (LogMAR)
Antonios et al. (2015)	30	TICL	2°	−6.96 ± 3.68	−0.83 ± 0.76	0	0.17 ± 0.06	0.11 ± 0.05
Alfonso et al. (2010)	30	TICL	1°	−5.38 ± 3.26	−0.08 ± 0.37	0	0.1	0.1 ± 0.6
Abdelmassih et al. (2017)	16	TICL	2°	−7.34	−0.73	0	0.33	0.16
Budo et al. (2005)	6	Iris-fixated	1°	−13.88 sph −3.75 cyl	0.29 sph −1.33 cyl	0		
Venter (2009)	18	Iris-fixated	1°	−6.17	0.13	0	NA	NA
Güell et al. (2012)	17	Iris-fixated	2°	−6.99 ± 3.2	−0.22 ± 0.33	0	0.17 ± 0.13	0.10 ± 0.09
Current study, Eldanasoury et al. (2019)	50	ICL/TICL	1° and 2°	−5.85 D ± 4.14	−0.21 D ± 0.60	0	0.05 ± 0.12	−0.02 ± 0.09

# denotes number of eyes; pIOL denotes phakic intraocular lens; 1° denotes primary surgery; 2° denotes secondary surgery; pre-op denotes preoperative; post-op denotes postoperative; CDVA denotes corrected distance visual acuity; UDVA denotes uncorrected distance visual acuity; ICL denotes implantable collamer lens; TICL denotes toric implantable collamer lens; sph denotes sphere; cyl denotes cylinder

example, Alfonso et al. (2008) [26] reported no eyes lost two or more lines of CDVA similar to our experience. They [26, 30] concluded that the procedure was safe, efficacious, and predictable as a primary treatment of myopia and astigmatism associated with keratoconus. Budo et al. (2005) [31] initial evaluation of an iris-fixated pIOL as a primary procedure in keratoconus reported no loss of two or more lines of BCVA. More recently, Abdelmassih et al. (2017) [32] reported no loss of two or more lines of BCVA after sequential ICL implantation after intracorneal ring segment implantation and corneal cross-linking in keratoconic eyes.

Postoperative endothelial cell loss is a complication of pIOLs [17–20]. However, accurate preoperative measurement and selection of an appropriately sized pIOL can mitigate the risk of endothelial cell loss. In our study, endothelial cell counts decreased by 38 cells/mm^2 (-1.4%) from preoperatively to 1 year postoperatively. Güell et al. [27] reported a decrease of 13 cells/mm^2 (-0.5%) from preoperatively to 2 years postoperatively. Abdelmassih et al. (2017) [32] reported a loss of 256 cells/mm^2 (-8.89%) at 3 years postoperatively.

Phakic IOLs for keratoconus are a viable treatment for the correction of lower-order aberrations (sphere and cylinder) associated with keratoconus. However, higher-order aberrations remain after implantation, and patients should be advised that visual quality might still be less than desirable postoperatively. Ramin et al. (2018) [33] recent study reported no statistical change in corneal and internal higher-order aberrations (expect internal trefoil). Given that the majority of daily living visual tasks are dependent on lower-order aberrations, we believe that pIOL implantation increases the quality of life of keratoconus patients.

In summary, primary or secondary implantation of pIOLs for the correction of refractive error is a viable option in patients with stable keratoconus. Stable refractive outcomes, safety, and efficacy have been reported in a number of studies. However, many studies are limited due to a small sample size. We recommend adhering to stringent criteria for stability of the disease and a thorough assessment of any candidates prior to considering surgery.

References

1. Krachmer JH, Feder RS, Belin MW. Keratoconus and related noninflammatory corneal thinning disorders. Surv Ophthalmol. 1984;28(4):293–322.
2. Rabinowitz YS. Keratoconus. Surv Ophthalmol. 1998;42(4):297–319.
3. Godefrooij DA, de Wit GA, Uiterwaal CS, Imhof SM, Wisse RPL. Age-specific incidence and prevalence of keratoconus: a nationwide registration study. Am J Ophthalmol. 2017;175:169–72.
4. Hashemi H, Heydarian S, Yekta A, et al. High prevalence and familial aggregation of keratoconus in an Iranian rural population: a population-based study. Ophthalmic Physiol Opt. 2018;38:447–55.
5. Al-Bdour MD, Al-Till MI, Abu Khader IB. Causes of blindness among adult Jordanians: a hospital-based study. Eur J Ophthalmol. 2002;12(1):5–10.
6. Shehadeh MM, Diakonis VF, Jalil SA, Younis R, Qadoumi J, Al-Labadi L. Prevalence of keratoconus among a Palestinian tertiary student population. Open Ophthalmol J. 2015;9:172–6. https://doi.org/10.2174/1874364101509010172. [PMC free article] [PubMed] [CrossRef] [Google Scholar]

7. Abu-Amero KK, Al-Muammar AM, Kondkar AA. Genetics of keratoconus: where do we stand? J Ophthalmol. 2014;2014:641708.
8. Wilson SE, Klyce SD. Screening for corneal topographic abnormalities before refractive surgery. Ophthalmology. 1994;101:147–52.
9. Randleman JB, Dupps WJ Jr, Santhiago MR, Rabinowitz YS, Koch DD, Stulting RD, Klyce SD. Screening for keratoconus and related ectatic corneal disorders. Cornea. 2015;34(8):e20–2.
10. Klyce SD, Karon MD, Smolek MK. Screening patients with the corneal navigator. J Refract Surg. 2005;21:S617–22.
11. Shah S, Naroo S, Hosking S, Gherghel D, Mantry S, Bannerjee S, Pedwell K, Bains HS. Nidek OPD-scan analysis of normal, keratoconic, and penetrating keratoplasty eyes. J Refract Surg. 2003;19(2 Suppl):S255–9.
12. Amsler M. Le keratocone fruste au javal. Ophtalmologica. 1938;96:77–83.
13. Amsler M. Keratocone classique et keratocone fruste, arguments unitaires. Ophtalmologica. 1946;111:96–101.
14. Andreanos KD, Hashemi K, Petrelli M, Droutsas K, Georgalas I, Kymionis GD. Keratoconus treatment algorithm. Ophthalmol Therapy. 2017;6(2):245–62.
15. Caporossi A, Mazzotta C, Baiocchi S, Caporossi T. Long- term results of riboflavin ultraviolet a corneal collagen cross-linking for keratoconus in Italy: the Siena eye cross study. Am J Ophthalmol. 2010;149(4):585–93.
16. Vega-Estrada A, Alio JL. The use of intracorneal ring segments in keratoconus. Eye Vis (Lond). 2016;3(8) https://doi.org/10.1186/s40662-016-0040-z. eCollection 2016. Review.
17. Alió JL, Peña-García P, Abdulla GF, Zein G, Abu-Mustafa SK. Comparison of iris-claw and posterior chamber collagen copolymer phakic intraocular lenses in keratoconus. J Cataract Refract Surg. 2014;40(3):383–94.
18. Fechner PU, van der Heijde GL, Worst JG. Intraocular lens for the correction of myopia of the phakic eye. Klin Monatsbl Augenheilkd. 1988;193:29–34.
19. Fechner PU, Singh D, Wulff K. Iris-claw lens in phakic eyes to correct hyperopia: preliminary study. J Cataract Refract Surg. 1998;24:48–56.
20. Fechner PU, Haubitz I, Wichmann W, Wulff K. Worst- Fechner biconcave minus power phakic iris-claw lens. J Refract Surg. 1999;15:93–105.
21. Kamiya K, Shimizu K, Ando W, Asato Y, Fujisawa T. Phakic toric implantable collamer lens implantation for the correction of high myopic astigmatism in eyes with keratoconus. J Refract Surg. 2008;24:840–2.
22. Boxer Wachler BS, Vicente LL. Optimizing the vault of collagen copolymer phakic intraocular lenses in eyes with keratoconus and myopia: comparison of 2 methods. J Cataract Refract Surg. 2010;36:1741–4.
23. Nakamura T, Isogai N, Kojima T, Yoshida Y, Sugiyama Y. Implantable collamer lens sizing method based on swept-source anterior segment optical coherence tomography. Am J Ophthalmol. 2018;187:99–107.
24. Kanellopoulos J, Asimellis G. Keratoconus management: long-term stability of topography-guided normalization combined with high-fluence CXL stabilization (the Athens protocol). J Refract Surg. 2014;30:88–93.
25. Iqbal M, Elmassry A, Tawfik A, Elgharieb ME, El Deen Al Nahrawy OM, Soliman AH, Saad HA, Ibrahim Elzembely HA, Saeed AM, Mohammed OA, Kamel AG, El Saman IS. Evaluation of the effectiveness of cross-linking combined with photorefractive keratectomy for treatment of keratoconus. Cornea. 2018;37(9):1143–50.
26. Alfonso JF, Palacios A, Montés-Micó R. Myopic phakic STAAR collamer posterior chamber intraocular lenses for keratoconus. J Refract Surg. 2008;24(9):867–74.
27. Antonios R, Dirani A, Fadlallah A, Chelala E, Hamade A, Cherfane C, Jarade E. Safety and visual outcome of visian toric ICL implantation after corneal collagen cross-linking in keratoconus: up to 2 years of follow-up. J Ophthalmol. 2015;2015:514834.

28. Güell JL, Morral M, Malecaze F, Gris O, Elies D, Manero F. Collagen crosslinking and toric iris-claw phakic intraocular lens for myopic astigmatism in progressive mild to moderate keratoconus. J Cataract Refract Surg. 2012;38(3):475–84.
29. Venter J. Artisan phakic intraocular lens in patients with keratoconus. J Refract Surg. 2009;25(9):759–64.
30. Alfonso JF, Fernández-Vega L, Lisa C, Fernandes P, González-Méijome JM, Montés-Micó R. Collagen copolymer toric posterior chamber phakic intraocular lens in eyes with keratoconus. J Cataract Refract Surg. 2010;36(6):906–16.
31. Budo C, Bartels MC, van Rij G. Implantation of Artisan toric phakic intraocular lenses for the correction of astigmatism and spherical errors in patients with keratoconus. J Refract Surg. 2005;21(3):218–22.
32. Abdelmassih Y, El-Khoury S, Chelala E, Slim E, Cherfan CG, Jarade E. Toric ICL implantation after sequential intracorneal ring segments implantation and corneal cross-linking in keratoconus: 2-year follow-up. J Refract Surg. 2017;33(9):610–6.
33. Ramin S, Sangin Abadi A, Doroodgar F, Esmaeili M, Niazi F, Niazi S, Alinia C, Golestani Y, Taj AR. Comparison of visual, refractive and aberration measurements of INTACS versus toric ICL lens implantation; a four-year follow-up. Med Hypothesis Disov Innov Ophthalmol. 2018;7(1):32–9.

Excimer Laser and Keratoconus

César Carriazo and María José Cosentino

One may well wonder when it is possible to perform an excimer laser surgery in a patient with keratoconus: which should be ideally carried out in a patient who wants to be visually rehabilitated and who has irregular astigmatism and contact lens intolerance. Which is the aim of this? The aim of this is both to improve the visual quality and reduce ghost images, which may even secondarily improve the uncorrected visual acuity [1–15].

It is important to meet the inclusion criteria to ensure the satisfaction of the procedure. Within those criteria, we have to mention the stable refraction for at least 1 year, the corneal topography without changes for at least 18 months, and the patient's age over 35 years.

Therefore, it will be convenient to look for an alternative treatment technique when every patient presents unstable refraction, corneal topography with changes within a period less than 18 months, keratometries higher than 49 D, residual pachymetry after ablation with excimer laser less than 400 microns, and under 35 years of age.

We carefully studied 28 cases with mild keratoconus or in keratoconus suspicious cases, whose characteristics were present in the abovementioned criteria of inclusion. The inferior-superior asymmetry was of 1.71, with an age average of 42.5 ± 3.1 years, taking into account the analyzed population, after 16 years of the procedure. The preoperative spherical equivalent was −4.77 ± 1.43 diopters, with a spherical component of − 4.18 diopters and a cylindrical component of −1.31

Electronic Supplementary Material The online version of this chapter (https://doi.org/10.1007/978-3-030-66143-4_8) contains supplementary material, which is available to authorized users.

C. Carriazo
Clínica Carriazo, Universidad del Norte, Barranquilla, Colombia

M. J. Cosentino (✉)
Instituto de la Vision, Universidad de Buenos Aires, Buenos Aires, Argentina

© Springer Nature Switzerland AG 2021
C. Carriazo, M. J. Cosentino (eds.), *New Frontiers for the Treatment of Keratoconus*, https://doi.org/10.1007/978-3-030-66143-4_8

diopters. The postoperative spherical equivalent was 0.66 ± 0.39 diopters, with a spherical component of −0.44 diopters and a cylindrical component of 0.5 diopters.

The preoperative best corrected visual acuity was 0.84 ± 0.13, and the postoperative one was 0.89 ± 0.21. All the cases were within 1 diopter of correction and 18 cases within 0.5 diopter of correction in the inmediate postoperative period. It should be noted regarding the security of the procedure that all the cases kept their best corrected visual acuity. The uncorrected distance visual acuity showed satisfactory results: 100% obtained 20/40 or more and 57.1% obtained 20/20 or more.

We believe the excimer laser can be a useful and secure tool for the cases of suspicious corneas and with low ametropia. What is important is the choice of criteria of the patients [16–30].

Over the last years, keratoconus has been treated with excimer laser although the corneas are weak and thin. This has even improved due to the fact we, nowadays, have cross-linking technology which has helped us stop a lot of keratoconus progression.

It is important to clarify that the surgery with excimer laser is a photorefractive and not a relaxing surgery, so its keratometry changes happen while the corneal structure keeps its structural strength since if it is lost by any pre-existing pathology or an excessive thinning, stromal weakening is induced and then corneal ectasia can be developed.

This means unlike the relaxing incisions (which have their keratometry changes by steepening the incised tissue which is relaxed and getting a distal flattening), the excimer laser does not look for relaxing the photorefractive tissue; on the contrary, it looks for a flattening, reducing the thickness of the treated area.

When we treat a cornea with keratoconus, we have to consider such cornea as a weak one per se. Thus, we have to take some aspects into consideration when we perform a photorefractive surgery in such corneas. Keratoconic corneas produce an asymmetric steepening at the expense of mainly thinning the cornea in the inferotemporal quadrant. The irregular astigmatism induced by the said pathology generally has an important myopic component. Therefore, if this is corrected by using the excimer laser, we have to compulsorily make a photorefractive surgery in the most curved point of the cornea which is very close to the thinnest one (besides, this may be the weakest point of this cornea).

On one hand, in Fig. 1, the customized profile which would use the laser for this case is observed. It can be observed that the larger ablation is produced in the most curved area of this cornea and, hence, in the thinnest and weakest point of the cornea.

On the other hand, as these cases are weak corneas – with or without cross-linking – their response to curvature change before a laser ablation is not going to have the same predictability that we obtain in normal corneas. Moreover, this will depend on the amount of the ablated tissue. A worsening of the ectasia may be even induced [31–41].

Then, when we perform corneal remodeling in a keratoconic cornea, the annular or crescentic resection calculated for each patient is to aim at changing astigmatic vector and at getting it closer to emmetropia. Furthermore, in some cases, a small hyperopic component is left so that in the postoperative visual rehabilitation period, the programmed ablation will not be performed in the thinnest area of the cornea (in case of excimer laser need).

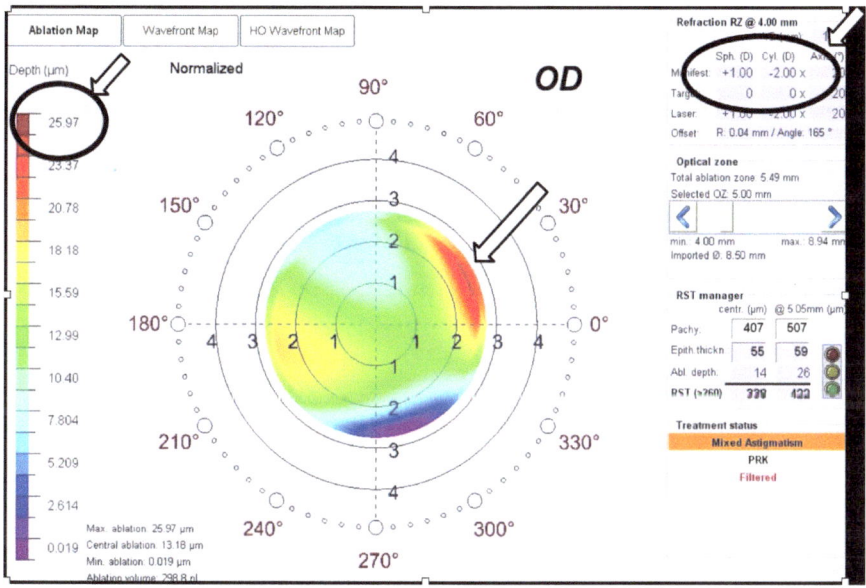

Fig. 1 Correction calculated by the aberrometry software to correct the coma plus 80% of the residual mixed astigmatism

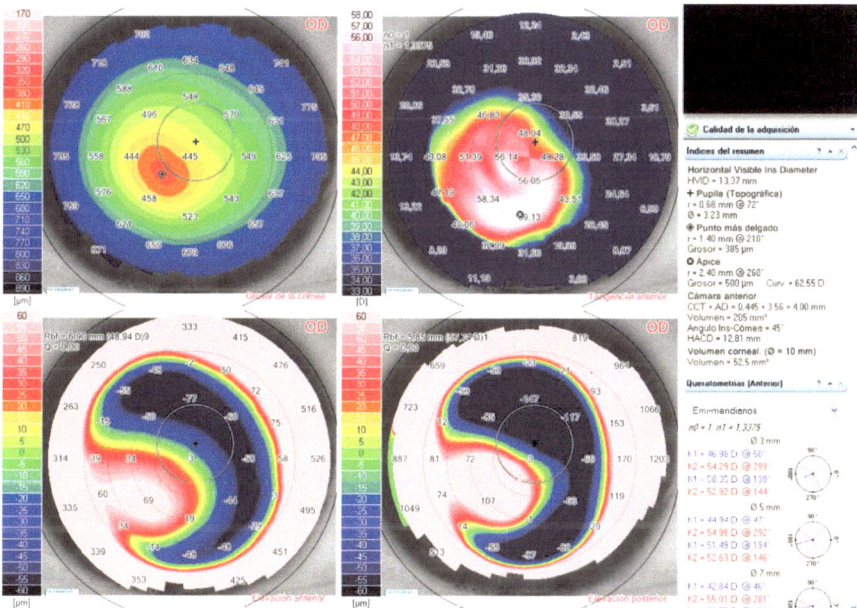

Fig. 2 Preoperative tomography of a patient with keratoconus

In Fig. 2, a profile which would be used if this cornea with keratoconus was treated with excimer laser before being treated with corneal remodeling technique is shown, and in Fig. 3, the profile of the suitable treatment in the said cornea after

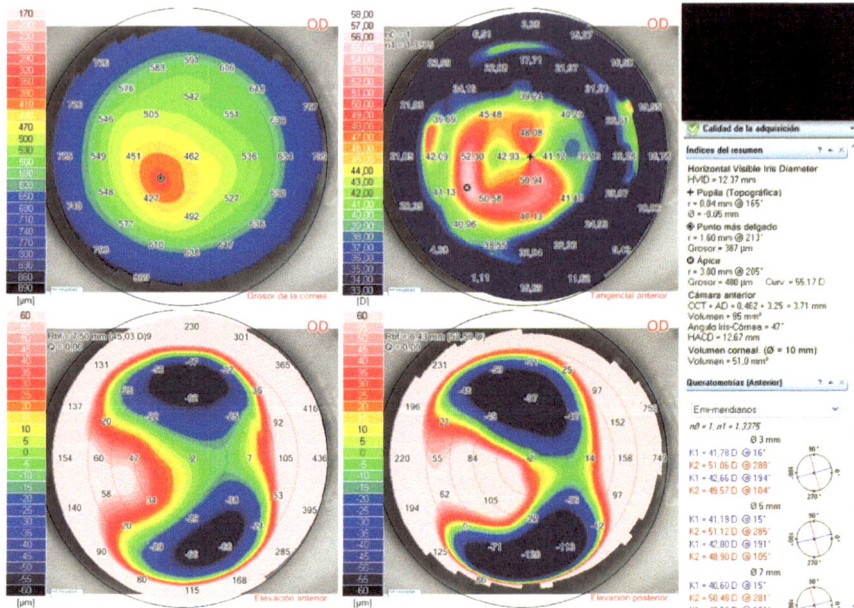

Fig. 3 Postoperative corneal tomography of the same keratoconus case in Figure 2 treated with the Corneal Remodeling technique

the corneal remodeling technique can be observed. In the first case, it can be seen how the larger ablation is performed in the most curved and thinnest point of the cornea, and in the second one, one can note how excimer laser ablation avoids removing the tissue in the thinnest point of the cornea. The reason is that this point changed from a curved and weak into a flat and not so weak area (after the vector change produced by the corneal remodeling technique previously performed). That offers us greater reliability in the postoperative biomechanical behavior of this type of patients.

When we reflect on corneal biomechanics, it does not mean that we disagree about performing PRK (photorefractive keratectomy) in some patients with keratoconus. On the contrary, we think the excimer laser is a very useful tool to treat these patients but under some considerations.

We believe that the excimer laser is a useful and reliable tool for cases of suspicious corneas and with low ametropia. We compared with a similar population of patients where surface ablation was performed associated with cross-linking (but with less follow-up), and the results did not show statistically significant differences.

We consider if a surface ablation in a keratoconus is performed, such ablation must be always done as long as it is a forme fruste or stage 1 keratoconus, related to low refractive errors. If they were more advanced-stage keratoconus or keratoconus with high refractive errors, they would have to be necessarily treated with high ablations which would further weaken the cornea.

Furthermore, these ablations must be accompanied with previous treatments or together with cross-linking. An important consideration when programming the patient's correction jointly with cross-linking is our target must be toward a low residual myopia since the cross-linking may induce corneal flattening per se.

On the other hand, if we treat keratoconus in more advanced stages with excimer laser, we will not obtain postoperative good visual quality. Although they can improve preoperative vision, this should definitely not be an indication for performing excimer laser in this kind of stages: nowadays, we do not recommend treating stage 2 or higher stages of keratoconus with excimer laser.

Finally, we must take into account that when we implant intracorneal rings or perform corneal remodeling technique, we will always have some degree of irregular astigmatism, which makes it mandatory to use wavefront technology with excimer laser to correct these aberrations. The high-order aberration with the greatest visual impact is the coma, and it is the one we recommend to correct in these corneas which have received intracorneal ring implants or corneal remodeling.

To correct the coma, it is necessary to bear in mind that each case must be personalized, and one seeks to remove the least amount of tissue in the thinnest area of the cornea but with the greatest possible correction. This is achieved by reducing the optical zone, correcting the greatest possible coma, and calculating the impact of the coma correction on the defocus. Therefore, when we correct the entire coma, simultaneously, we should only partially correct the "defocus" since treating the entire coma inevitably has an impact on the defocus. For this reason, in some excimer laser manufacturers, if the entire coma is treated plus the entire defocus, a hypercorrection can be obtained.

Ideally, the software incorporated into the excimer laser should calculate this impact on the defocus in order that this calculation is made automatically, which is not at least the case today in our technology.

With our excimer laser technology, we treat as much of the coma as possible using the transPRK module and only 80% of the patient's defocus. Although we know that with this method only a few cases achieve immediate emmetropia, in this way, we ensure that there are no hypercorrections and our results are very close to emmetropia, leaving our patients very happy.

This also leaves the door open for a "fine-tuning touch" after the result has been stabilized.

Customized Ablation in Patients with Post-intracorneal Ring Implantation and Corneal Remodeling

It must be taken into consideration that in a customized treatment – in which we correct coma and defocus – the greatest ablation must be done in the area of the cornea where there is the greatest thickness. In order to achieve this, we must understand the biomechanical response of the cornea and the target we must look for in the postoperative rings or corneal remodeling technique [42–45].

A great challenge for us, the refractive surgeons, is to be able to correct these patients operated of rings and corneal remodeling with the best result while we protect the corneal biomechanics.

In order to achieve this, whenever we perform these techniques, our target for each patient must be focused on leaving a refractive defect close to the emmetropia but with a residual defocus, which allows its correction without mostly weakening the thinnest part of the cornea.

It is very important to explain that it is not the same to treat the coma in a cornea after intracorneal rings or after corneal remodeling technique with a neutral subjective refraction as a case with myopic or hyperopic astigmatism.

Figure 1 shows the correction calculated by the aberrometry software to correct the coma plus 80% of the residual mixed astigmatism. Figure 2 shows the preoperative tomography of a patient with keratoconus, and Fig. 3 shows the Fig. 4. Postoperative corneal tomography of residual astigmatism after Corneal Remodeling technique regularized by excimer laser which was performed in 2015. A corneal flattening greater than 7 diopters is observed. Likewise, Fig. 4 shows the postoperative period where the patient's astigmatism is regularized.

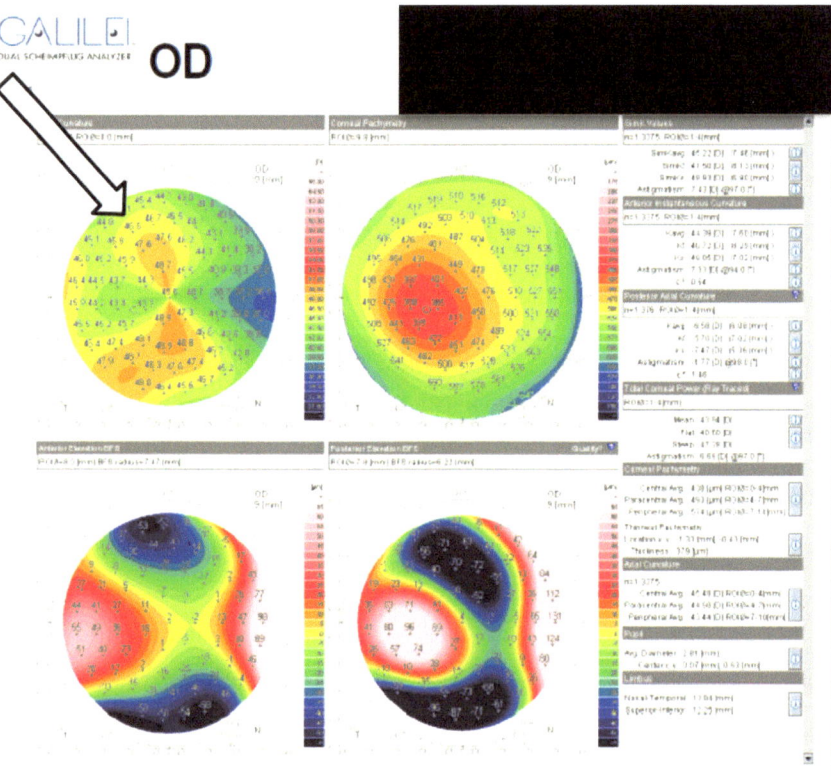

Fig. 4 Postoperative astigmatism regularized by excimer laser

In Fig. 5a, b, in the simulation, we show the difference that there is in the correction of mixed astigmatism compared to a myopic compound astigmatism. Figure 5a shows the guided ablation map calculated by the aberrometry software to correct this coma plus 80% of its mixed astigmatism defect. Figure 5b shows the guided ablation map calculated by the aberrometry software to correct this same coma but

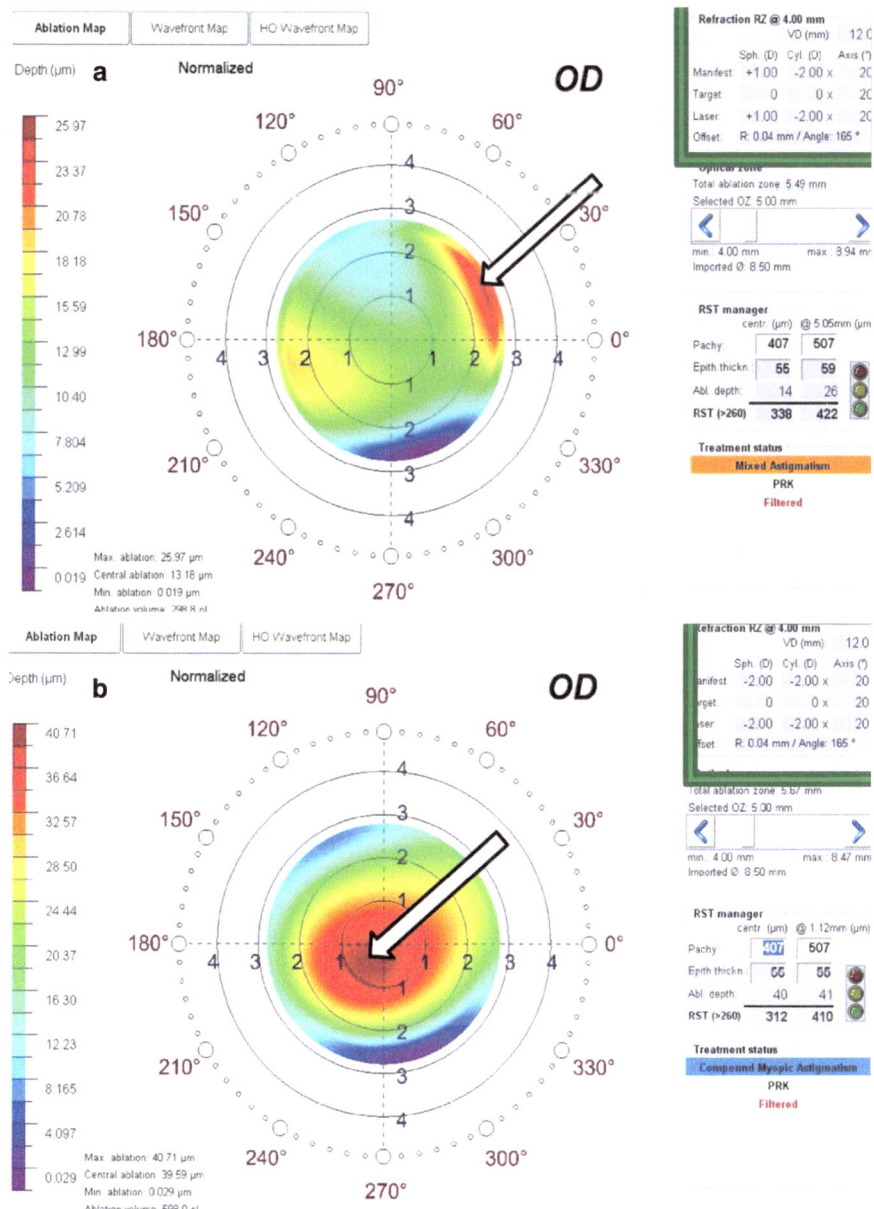

Fig. 5 (**a, b**) Simulation about correction of mixed astigmatism compared to a myopic compound astigmatism

with a simulated myopic astigmatism defect. It can be seen that in the last case, the thinnest and weakest part of the cornea is largely ablated.

Video 1 shows customized PRK performed in a keratoconic cornea.

To conclude, it is important to highlight that if we want to protect a cornea with keratoconus and refractive defects (except in presbyopic patients that we want to get some monovision), the ideal situation is to consider corneal remodeling technique with a slightly expected hyperopic or mixed astigmatism target to conserve the obtained improvement of corneal biomechanics.

References

1. Bardan AS, Lee H, Nanavaty MA. Outcomes of simultaneous and sequential cross-linking with excimer laser. J Refract Surg. 2018;34(10):690–6.
2. Müller TM, Lange AP. Topography-guided PRK and crosslinking in eyes with keratoconus and post-LASIK ectasia. Klin Monbl Augenheilkd. 2017;234(4):451–4. 28192838.
3. Pahuja NK, Shetty R, Sinha Roy A, Thakkar MM, Jayadev C, Nuijts RM, Nagaraja H. Laser vision correction with Q factor modification for keratoconus management. Curr Eye Res. 2017;42(4):542–8.
4. Fung SS, Aiello F, Maurino V. Outcomes of femtosecond laser-assisted mushroom-configuration keratoplasty in advanced keratoconus. Eye (Lond). 2016;30(4):553–61. https://doi.org/10.1038/eye.2015.273. Epub 2016 Jan 22
5. Kanellopoulos AJ, Asimellis G. Novel placido-derived topography-guided excimer corneal normalization with cyclorotation adjustment: enhanced Athens protocol for keratoconus. J Refract Surg. 2015 Nov;31(11):768–73.
6. Donoso R, Díaz C, Villavicencio P. Long-term results of lasik refractive error correction after penetrating keratoplasty in patients with keratoconus. Arch Soc Esp Oftalmol. 2015;90(7):308–11.
7. Wu W, Wang Y, Xu L. Meta-analysis of Pentacam vs. ultrasound pachymetry in central corneal thickness measurement in normal, post-LASIK or PRK, and keratoconic or keratoconus-suspect eyes.
8. Kanellopoulos AJ, Asimellis G. Comparison of Placido disc and Scheimpflug image-derived topography-guided excimer laser surface normalization combined with higher fluence CXL: the Athens Protocol, in progressive keratoconus. Clin Ophthalmol. 2013;7:1385–96.
9. Yam JC, Cheng AC. Prognostic factors for visual outcomes after crosslinking for keratoconus and post-LASIK ectasia. Eur J Ophthalmol. 2013;23(6):799–806.
10. Elsahn AF, Rapuano CJ, Antunes VA, Abdalla YF, Cohen EJ. Excimer laser phototherapeutic keratectomy for keratoconus nodules. Cornea. 2009;28(2):144–7.
11. Tan BU, Purcell TL, Torres LF, Schanzlin DJ. New surgical approaches to the management of keratoconus and post-LASIK ectasia. Trans Am Ophthalmol Soc. 2006;104:212–20.
12. Binder PS, Lindstrom RL, Stulting RD, Donnenfeld E, Wu H, McDonnell P, Rabinowitz Y. Keratoconus and corneal ectasia after LASIK. J Cataract Refract Surg. 2005;31(11):2035–8. No abstract available
13. Kasparova EA, Kasparov AA. Six-year experience with excimer laser surgery for primary keratoconus in Russia. J Refract Surg. 2003;19(2 Suppl):S250–4.
14. Al-Mohaimeed MM. Combined corneal CXL and photorefractive keratectomy for treatment of keratoconus: a review. Al-Mohaimeed MM Int J Ophthalmol. 2019;12(12):1929–38.
15. Kymionis GD, Grentzelos MA, Voulgari N. Stromal scarring and visual acuity loss after combined PRK and CXL for keratoconus. J Refract Surg. 2019;35(6):399.

16. Kanellopoulos AJ. The impact of keratoconus treatment with the Athens Protocol (partial topography-guided photorefractive keratectomy combined with higher-fluence corneal collagen cross-linking) on quality of life: a long-term study. Clin Ophthalmol. 2019;13:795–803.

17. Kanellopoulos AJ. Management of progressive keratoconus with partial topography-guided PRK combined with refractive, customized CXL – a novel technique: the enhanced Athens protocol.

18. Moraes RLB, Ghanem RC, Ghanem VC, Santhiago MR. Haze and visual acuity loss after sequential photorefractive keratectomy and corneal cross-linking for keratoconus. J Refract Surg. 2019;35(2):109–14.

19. Iqbal M, Elmassry A, Tawfik A, Elgharieb M, Nagy K, Soliman A, Saad H, Tawfik T, Ali O, Gad A, El Saman I, Radwan A, Elzembely H, Abou Ali A, Fawzy O. Standard cross-linking versus photorefractive keratectomy combined with accelerated cross-linking for keratoconus management: a comparative study. Acta Ophthalmol. 2019;97(4):e623–31.

20. Abou Samra W, Mokbel T, Elwan M, Saleh S, Elwehidy A, Iqbal M, Ellayeh A. Two-stage procedure in the management of selected cases of keratoconus: clear lens extraction with aspherical IOL implantation followed by WFG-PRK. Int J Ophthalmol. 2018;11(11):1761–7.

21. Gore DM, Leucci MT, Anand V, Fernandez-Vega Cueto L, Arba Mosquera S, Allan BD. Combined wavefront-guided transepithelial photorefractive keratectomy and corneal crosslinking for visual rehabilitation in moderate keratoconus. J Cataract Refract Surg. 2018;44(5):571–80. https://doi.org/10.1016/j.jcrs.2018.03.026.

22. Al-Amri AM. 5-year follow-up of combined non-topography guided photorefractive keratectomy and corneal collagen cross linking for keratoconus. Int J Ophthalmol. 2018;11(1):48–52.

23. Grentzelos MA, Kounis GA, Diakonis VF, Siganos CS, Tsilimbaris MK, Pallikaris IG, Kymionis GD. Combined transepithelial phototherapeutic keratectomy and conventional photorefractive keratectomy followed simultaneously by corneal crosslinking for keratoconus: cretan protocol plus. J Cataract Refract Surg. 2017;43(10):1257–62.

24. Müller TM, Lange AP. Topography-guided PRK and crosslinking in eyes with keratoconus and post-LASIK ectasia. Klin Monatsbl Augenheilkd. 2017;234(4):451–4.

25. Sakla H, Altroudi W, Munoz G, Sakla Y. Simultaneous topography-guided photorefractive keratectomy and accelerated corneal collagen cross-linking for keratoconus. Cornea. 2016;35(7):941–5.

26. Al-Tuwairqi WS, Osuagwu UL, Razzouk H, Ogbuehi KC. One-year clinical outcomes of a two-step surgical management for keratoconus-topography-guided photorefractive keratectomy/cross-linking after intrastromal corneal ring implantation. Eye Contact Lens. 2015;41(6):359–66.

27. Khakshoor H, Razavi F, Eslampour A, Omdtabrizi A. Photorefractive keratectomy in mild to moderate keratoconus: outcomes in over 40-year-old patients. Indian J Ophthalmol. 2015;63(2):157–61.

28. Fadlallah A, Dirani A, Chelala E, Antonios R, Cherfan G, Jarade E. Non-topography-guided PRK combined with CXL for the correction of refractive errors in patients with early stage keratoconus. J Refract Surg. 2014;30(10):688–93.

29. Sakla H, Altroudi W, Muñoz G, Albarrán-Diego C. Simultaneous topography-guided partial photorefractive keratectomy and corneal collagen crosslinking for keratoconus. J Cataract Refract Surg. 2014;40(9):1430–8.

30. Dirani A, Fadlallah A, Syed ZA, Chelala E, Khoueir Z, Cherfan G, Jarade E. Non-topography-guided photorefractive keratectomy for the correction of residual mild refractive errors after ICRS implantation and CXL in keratoconus. J Refract Surg. 2014;30(4):266–71.

31. Wu W, Wang Y, Xu L. Meta-analysis of Pentacam vs. ultrasound pachymetry in central corneal thickness measurement in normal, post-LASIK or PRK, and keratoconic or keratoconus-suspect eyes. Graefes Arch Clin Exp Ophthalmol. 2014;252(1):91–9.

32. Alessio G, L'abbate M, Sborgia C, La Tegola MG. Photorefractive keratectomy followed by cross-linking versus cross-linking alone for management of progressive keratoconus: two-year follow-up. Am J Ophthalmol. 2013;155(1):54–65.e1.

33. Kremer I, Aizenman I, Lichter H, Shayer S, Levinger S. Simultaneous wavefront-guided photorefractive keratectomy and corneal collagen crosslinking after intrastromal corneal ring segment implantation for keratoconus. J Cataract Refract Surg. 2012;38(10):1802–7.
34. Tuwairqi WS, Sinjab MM. Safety and efficacy of simultaneous corneal collagen cross-linking with topography-guided PRK in managing low-grade keratoconus: 1-year follow-up. J Refract Surg. 2012;28(5):341–5.
35. Iovieno A, Légaré ME, Rootman DB, Yeung SN, Kim P, Rootman DS. Intracorneal ring segments implantation followed by same-day photorefractive keratectomy and corneal collagen cross-linking in keratoconus. J Refract Surg. 2011;27(12):915–8.
36. Spadea L. Collagen crosslinking for ectasia following PRK performed in excimer laser-assisted keratoplasty for keratoconus. Eur J Ophthalmol. 2012;22(2):274–7.
37. Koh IH, Seo KY, Park SB, Yang H, Kim I, Kim JS, Hwang DG, Nam SM. One-year efficacy and safety of combined photorefractive keratectomy and accelerated corneal collagen cross-linking after intacs SK intracorneal ring segment implantation in moderate keratoconus. Biomed Res Int. 2019;2019:7850216.
38. Rocha G, Ibrahim T, Gulliver E, Lewis K. Combined phototherapeutic keratectomy, intracorneal ring segment implantation, and corneal collagen cross-linking in keratoconus management. Cornea. 2019;38(10):1233–8.
39. Ahmet S, Ağca A, Yaşa D, Koç AA, Toğaç M, Yıldırım Y, Yıldız BK, Demirok A. Simultaneous transepithelial topography-guided photorefractive keratectomy and accelerated cross-linking in keratoconus: 2-year follow-up. Biomed Res Int. 2018;2018:2945751.
40. Sarac O, Kosekahya P, Caglayan M, Tanriverdi B, Taslipinar Uzel AG, Cagil N. Mechanical versus transepithelial phototherapeutic keratectomy epithelial removal followed by accelerated corneal crosslinking for pediatric keratoconus: long-term results. J Cataract Refract Surg. 2018;44(7):827–35.
41. Iqbal M, Elmassry A, Tawfik A, Elgharieb ME, El Deen Al Nahrawy OM, Soliman AH, Saad HA, Ibrahim Elzembely HA, Saeed AM, Mohammed OA, Kamel AG, El Saman IS. Evaluation of the effectiveness of cross-linking combined with photorefractive keratectomy for treatment of keratoconus. Cornea. 2018;37(9):1143–50.
42. Coskunseven E, Sharma DP, Grentzelos MA, Sahin O, Kymionis GD, Pallikaris I. Four-stage procedure for keratoconus: ICRS implantation, corneal cross-linking, toric phakic intraocular lens implantation, and topography-guided photorefractive keratectomy. J Refract Surg. 2017;33(10):683–9.
43. Chen X, Stojanovic A, Wang X, Liang J, Hu D, Utheim TP. Epithelial thickness profile change after combined topography-guided transepithelial photorefractive keratectomy and corneal cross-linking in treatment of keratoconus. J Refract Surg. 2016;32(9):626–34.
44. Shaheen MS, Shalaby Bardan A, Piñero DP, Ezzeldin H, El-Kateb M, Helaly H, Khalifa MA. Wave front-guided photorefractive keratectomy using a high-resolution aberrometer after corneal collagen cross-linking in keratoconus. Cornea. 2016;35(7):946–53.
45. Sherif AM, Ammar MA, Mostafa YS, Gamal Eldin SA, Osman AA. One-year results of simultaneous topography-guided photorefractive keratectomy and corneal collagen cross-linking in keratoconus utilizing a modern ablation software. J Ophthalmol. 2015;2015:321953.

Regenerative Therapies for Keratoconus

Jorge L. Alió del Barrio, Verónica Vargas, and Jorge L. Alió

Introduction

Tissue engineering is the branch of science which uses the combinations of cells, biomaterials, and physicochemical factors with the objective of improving or replacing any biological function of the organism, in our case the improvement, regeneration, or substitution of the corneal stroma functions.

The corneal stroma composes more than 90% of the corneal thickness, and its strength functions, transparency, and refraction are due to its complex anatomy and ultrastructure. The extracellular matrix of the corneal stroma is not only a simple superposition of collagen lamellae, but their molecules lay out in a very precise and exact way in which a minimum alteration leads to a loss of tissue transparency. It is composed of (A) collagen, which is more than 70% of the cornea's dry weight, being type I the most abundant (75%), followed by types VI (17%) and V (2%), and (B) proteoglycans, including keratan sulfate, chondroitin sulfate, and dermatan sulfate. Keratan sulfate is the most abundant (65%), and its core protein is composed of lumican, mimecan, and keratocan [1]. The latter is of special relevance due to the

Electronic Supplementary Material The online version of this chapter (https://doi.org/10.1007/978-3-030-66143-4_9) contains supplementary material, which is available to authorized users.

J. L. Alió del Barrio · J. L. Alió (✉)
Cornea, Cataract and Refractive Surgery Unit, Vissum Instituto Oftalmológico de Alicante, Alicante, Spain

Universidad Miguel Hernández, Alicante, Spain
e-mail: jlalio@vissum.com

V. Vargas
Innovation and Investigation Department, Vissum Instituto Oftalmológico de Alicante, Alicante, Spain

© Springer Nature Switzerland AG 2021
C. Carriazo, M. J. Cosentino (eds.), *New Frontiers for the Treatment of Keratoconus*, https://doi.org/10.1007/978-3-030-66143-4_9

fact that the corneal stroma is the only tissue in the entire organism in which kera-tocan is expressed; for this reason, keratocan is considered a specific marker of keratocyte differentiation in tissue engineering [2]. The cellular component of the corneal stroma only occupies 2–3% of the stromal volume, and the predominant cells are the keratocytes, which are mesenchymal cells derived from the neural crest, with a flattened aspect and stellate shape that lies between the collagen lamel-lae. Keratocytes have long processes, so they can communicate with each other through gap junctions, creating a tridimensional reticle that contains the extracel-lular matrix that they secrete. Keratocytes are quiescent in the normal cornea, but they are responsible for a slow and constant replacement of the stromal extracellular matrix through the production of collagen, proteoglycans, glycosaminoglycans, and metalloproteinases, which are essential for a long-term maintenance of corneal transparency. When the cornea is wounded, keratocytes become metabolically active, and they differentiate into fibroblasts and myofibroblasts, which participate in stromal healing and subsequent production of opacities as a consequence of the loss of normal extracellular matrix ultrastructure.

Keratocytes are not only necessary for stromal remodeling; they also produce paracrine mediators which stablish epithelial-stromal interactions that are necessary for proliferation, motility, and differentiation of epithelial cells [3].

The renewal ability of stromal keratocytes was in doubt until a few years ago when their progenitor cells were localized in the anterior limbal corneal stroma (near the stem cells of the corneal epithelium), which express markers of adult stem cells like ABCG2 (ATP-binding cassette G2) and PAX6 (paired box 6) [4].

During the last decades, various attempts have been made, with greater or lesser success, to replicate the corneal stroma in the laboratory, in order to have artificial substitutes that could reduce or avoid the necessity of donor corneas [5].

Nevertheless, the high complexity of this tissue makes these artificial materials end up failing, either for a lack of transparency, an insufficient rigidity and consis-tence, or a poor capacity of integration with the in vivo surrounding tissue (and therefore its extrusion).

Due to the inability to artificially reproduce the corneal stroma in the laboratory, the idea of using ocular or extraocular stem cells has gained interest during the past years. These stem cells would differentiate into adult functional keratocytes, which will be able to produce in a natural way this complex tissue that is really hard to reproduce artificially.

Stem Cells Used in Corneal Stroma Tissue Engineering (Table 1) [1]

- Corneal stromal stem cells (CSSCs)
- Bone marrow mesenchymal stem cells (BM-MSCs)
- Adipose-derived adult stem cells (ADASCs) (Fig. 1a)

Table 1 Stem cells used in the corneal stromal regeneration. Evidence of their keratocyte differentiation capacity and their possible autologous use

	CSSC	BM-MSC	ADASC	UCMSC	ESC	iPSC
Differentiation keratocytic in vitro proven	Yes	Yes	Yes	Yes	Yes	Yes
Differentiation keratocytic in vivo proven	Yes	Yes	Yes	Yes	No	No
Possible autologous use	No	Yes	Yes	Yes/no	No	Yes

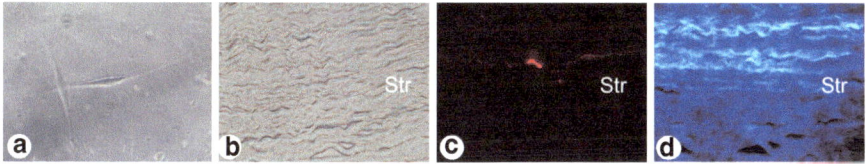

Fig. 1 Transplant of human ADASCs in rabbit stroma in vivo. (**a**) Culture of human ADASCs. (**b**) Phase-contrast photographs with morphologically intact stroma 3 months after transplantation. (**c**) Same section showing the survival of implanted cells labeled with Vybrant CM-DiL. (**d**) Same section showing the expression of new human collagen type I inside rabbit stroma (Str: stroma; 400× magnification). (Courtesy of Dr. Arnalich Montiel)

- Umbilical cord mesenchymal stem cells (UCMSCs)
- Embryonic stem cells (ESCs)
- Induced pluripotent stem cells (iPSCs)

All mesenchymal stem cells seem to have a similar in vivo behavior, being capable to differentiate into functional adult keratocytes and modulate the corneal stroma, showing immunomodulating properties that avoid any type of inflammatory response or rejection even in xenogeneic scenarios (interspecies).

Probably, the CSSCs have some advantages over the other cells due to the fact that they are corneal cells with a forthright differentiation potential. Nevertheless, the number of human stromal stem cells that can be obtained from each donor cornea is limited, which is technically challenging, and it is impossible to obtain them without damaging irreversibly the donor tissue. These are important limitations which make difficult their autologous use. Therefore the necessity to provide an alternative source of extraocular stem cells with keratocyte differentiation potential that could substitute the CSSCs in the corneal stromal tissue engineering.

The adipose human tissue has proven to be an ideal source of autologous stem cells, as it satisfies all requirements: it has an easy access, has high cellular efficiency, is easy to cultivate, and has stem cells' abilities; the ADASCs can differentiate into multiple cellular lines (keratocytes, osteoblasts, chondroblasts, myoblasts, hepatocytes, neurons, etc.) [1].

The differentiation into each cellular line occurs due to the environment and stimulating factors that are specific for each cell type, avoiding the mixture of different cell niches.

The BM-MSCs are very similar to the ADASCs, but their extraction requires a medullar puncture, which is a more complex and painful procedure requiring general anesthesia (the adipose tissue sample is generally obtained from the gluteal fat or lower back under local anesthesia). The UCMSCs are an attractive alternative, but their autologous use would require tissue banks in order to preserve the umbilical cord from birth for the entire population, which has a high cost and currently very few people own. The use of embryonic cells has been abandoned due to the ethical problems involved with their use but especially to the emergence of iPSCs [6], which do not present these problems since they derive from adult cells.

In 2012, the Japanese Shinya Yamanaka and the British John B. Gurdon received the medicine Nobel Prize for discovering that specialized mature cells can reprogram into immature cells or stem cells, with a capacity of differentiation into almost any cellular line in the organism. iPSCs promise to be the future of tissue and cellular engineering, and different lines of research are likely to derive from them in the coming years. As we have seen, stem cells have the potential of differentiation into adult keratocytes.

Nevertheless, it is important to consider that the possible therapeutic effect of stem cells in damaged tissue is not exclusive of their differentiation potential in the receptive tissue but to multiple mechanisms of action that contribute simultaneously, for example, the paracrine secretion of growth factors (like vascular endothelial growth factor (VEGF), platelet-derived growth factor (PDGF), hepatocyte growth factor (HGF), and transforming growth factor beta 1 (TGFβ1)) which have the capacity to stimulate dysfunctional host cells, reduce tissue damage, or activate immunomodulating responses, being the differentiation of MSCs, sometimes, non-relevant for the therapeutic effect or even inexistent [7–9].

Therapeutic Techniques Used in Corneal Stroma Tissue Engineering

Different in vivo techniques have been proposed and developed in order to transplant stem cells, with the objective to find the most appropriate method to regenerate the corneal stroma.

Stem Cell Implant in the Ocular Surface

This would be the ideal method to repair the ocular surface and regenerate the corneal epithelium in limbal deficiency cases. However, the superficial implantation of MSCs might be relevant for the prevention and modulation of anterior stromal scars. As we have mentioned, MSCs produce paracrine factors which promote corneal epithelial regeneration and stromal remodeling [10]. Therefore, the benefit of stem cells in the ocular surface could be more in relation with this paracrine effect than with the differentiation of these cells into corneal epithelial cells; this scientific evidence is controversial.

Di et al. studied subconjunctival injections of BM-MSCs in diabetic mice, reporting an increase in epithelial proliferation and an attenuation in the inflammatory response [11]. A study reported one case of a neurotrophic ulcer that was resistant to conventional treatment and healed with the topical application of autologous ADASC [12]. However, there is a lack of new clinical studies since 2012 which doubts its real efficacy. Finally, Basu et al. suggest the application of MSCs through the use of fibrin glue [13]. These authors showed in an animal model that CSSCs embedded in a fibrin human gel and polymerized by the addition of thrombin are capable of preventing stromal scarring after injury, in addition to generating new organized collagen equivalent to the receptors' tissue. Nowadays, this group is doing a clinical essay in humans in order to validate these results, using autologous and heterologous CSSCs obtained from limbal biopsies in cases of neurotrophic ulcers and ocular caustications. Its preliminary results are encouraging, showing an improvement in corneal epithelization and transparency [14].

Intrastromal Stem Cell Implantation

The direct implantation of stem cells in the corneal stroma has been used in vivo by several authors, to date only in animal experimentation models, showing the differentiation of different types of injected stem cells into adult and functional keratocytes, without any inflammatory response or rejection.

Our group was the first one to show the ADASC differentiation capacity in vivo and its capacity of producing a new human extracellular matrix inside the rabbit's cornea [15] (Fig. 1). This implantation is usually done through manually dissected intrastromal pockets or assisted with femtosecond laser.

Du et al. published the recovery of corneal thickness and transparency in lumican knockout mice (an animal model of corneal dystrophy which generates thin corneas, haze, and a stromal disorganization) 3 months after the implantation of human intrastromal CSSCs. They also showed the production of human keratan sulfate in the mouse stroma and a reorganization of the collagen receptor lamellae, concluding that CSSC transplant in human corneal stroma could alleviate the severity of preexisting leukomas without the need of any other surgical intervention [16]. Similar observations were reported by Liu et al. using UCMSCs in the same animal model [17]. Also, Thomas et al. observed that UCMSCs transplanted in the corneal stroma of a mouse model for mucopolysaccharidosis not only had a role in the digestion of accumulated extracellular glycosaminoglycans but they even allow (through a paracrine action) the participation of the hosts' dysfunctional keratocytes in this catabolism [18].

Our research team published in 2017 the first clinical essay in humans using stem cells with the objective of regenerating the corneal stroma [19]. In this small pilot study ($n = 5$), autologous ADASCs were transplanted (Fig. 2), obtained through elective liposuction, into an intrastromal pocket assisted with femtosecond laser in patients with advanced keratoconus (stage ≥ 4) whose only therapeutic alternative

Fig. 2 Microscopy appearance of human ADASCs (phase-contrast photography) prior to in vivo transplant (10×, magnification)

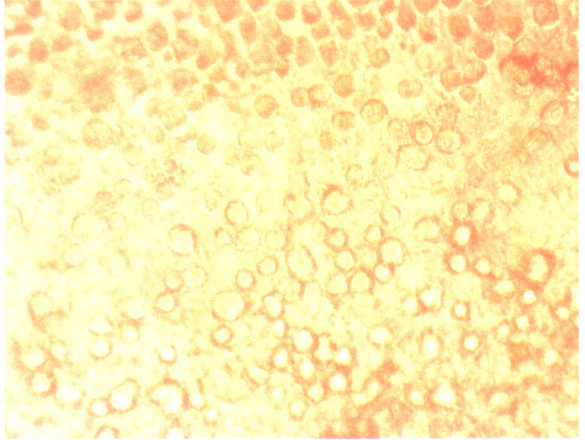

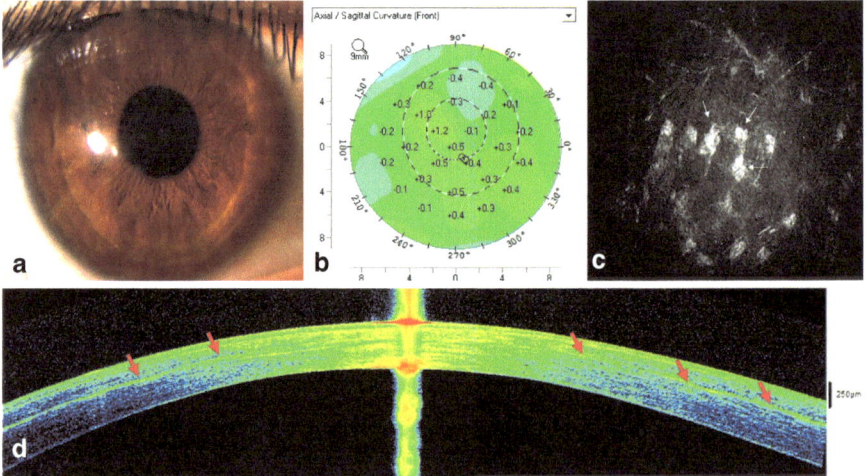

Fig. 3 Intrastromal transplant of human autologous ADASCs in patients with severe keratoconus. (**a**) Slit lamp image after 1-year follow-up. (**b**) Topographic changes between pre-op and 12 months after transplantation. There is a keratometric stability. (**c**) Confocal microscopy photos at surgical plane level 1 month after transplant. Cellular presence is confirmed by the presence of cells with round nucleus (white arrows) (the image corresponds to a 100 × 100 μm area). (**d**) Anterior segment OCT 1 year after transplant. Observe the patchy areas at the implantation level compatible with areas of new collagen production

was a corneal transplant (Video 1). We showed a modest gain in visual acuity, between one and two lines of vision, as well as cellular survival in vivo through confocal microscopy (Fig. 3c), the absence of any associated inflammatory response (Fig. 3a), and the emergence of small amounts of new-formed collagen, resulting in a slight increase in pachymetry (mean of 15 microns 1 year after surgery) (Fig. 3d). We could also appreciate the improvement of preexisting anterior stromal leukomas in one case [19].

Nowadays, it has been proven by our group and by other researchers that the production of human extracellular matrix by any of the mesenchymal stem cells occurs in vivo, but in small amounts, the reason why (in our opinion), quantitatively, it would not be enough to rehabilitate the thickness of a very thin or weak cornea, like in keratoconus. In these cases, it would be necessary to add a substrate to enhance or complement these results. On the other hand, the existing evidence in animal experimentation models suggests that the direct transplant of intrastromal stem cells might be a promising therapy in patients that have corneal dystrophies and progressive corneal opacifications in systemic metabolic diseases and in stromal scars.

Implantation of Intrastromal Stem Cells with a Biodegradable Scaffold

In order to boost the growth and survival of implanted stem cells into the corneal stroma, the addition of biodegradable synthetic extracellular matrixes along the cellular component has been studied. Espandar et al. transplanted human ADASCs along with a semi-solid hydrogel of hyaluronic acid inside the rabbit cornea, seeing a greater survival and keratocyte differentiation of ADASCs in comparison to those cases that had cellular transplant alone [20]. Ma et al. used rabbits' ADASCs with a biodegradable polylactic-co-glycolic acid (PLGA) as a scaffold, with similar results [21].

Implantation of Intrastromal Stem Cells with No Biodegradable Scaffold

The main obstacle for the production of an artificial cornea is the reproduction of the stromal architecture; this is why it has not been possible to generate clinically viable synthetic corneal equivalents for use in humans. Most of these stromal analogous created so far consists in human keratocytes cultured in collagen-based materials, with the objective that once they have been implanted, they can be remodeled [4].

New and improved biomaterials compatible with the human cornea have been developed recently, like poly(methyl methacrylate) hydrogels, collagen-chondroitin sulfate hydrogels, and polyurethanes [22].

The combination of these biomaterials with cells could generate promising equivalents of the stroma, and a few studies have been published in which the adult corneal cells are used (including keratocytes) with positive results regarding cellular adhesion and survival [23].

However, until now, few studies have been done in vivo, and there are not any studies that investigate the combinations of these synthetic stromal substitutes along with stem cells. Minura et al. used corneal fibroblast precursors along with porous gelatin hydrogels (in vivo, in an animal model), observing an intense expression of type I collagen. Nevertheless, these resulted to be weak and unstable, making impossible its clinical use [24].

Our research group has also investigated this possibility of stromal regeneration, analyzing the survival and biointegration of grafts composed of poly(ethyl acrylate) (PEA) macroporous membranes (Fig. 4a) colonized with ADASCs and transplanted in vivo inside the rabbit stroma (Fig. 4c) [25].

The hypothesis was that stem cells inside this porous material would differentiate into keratocytes and fill this porous material with corneal extracellular matrix that would allow a proper anchoring and integration of the synthetic material into the surrounding stroma. We could demonstrate the in vivo survival of ADASCs inside the synthetic grafts after 3-month follow-up (Fig. 4b), but not their proper differentiation into adult keratocytes nor a reduction in the extrusion rate of the implant (Fig. 4e). Our opinion is that stem cells do not receive a proper stimulus to differentiate into keratocytes in the presence of synthetic biomaterials, losing the chance to generate new collagen and therefore failing in the correct biointegration of the material (Fig. 4d), which finally ends up being extruded by the constant friction between the nonintegrated biomaterial and the surrounding stroma.

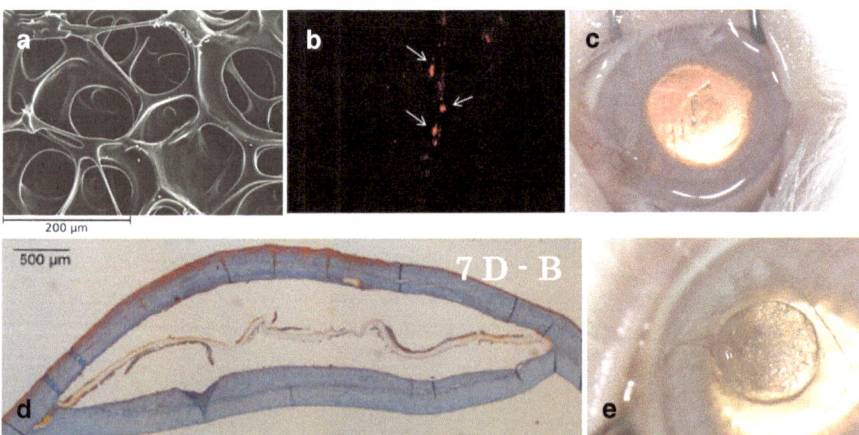

Fig. 4 Transplant of macroporous membranes of PEA along human ADASCs in the stromal in vivo model. (**a**) Image of electronic microscopy of PEA. (**b**) Cell survival at 3 months. (**c**) Intrastromal in vivo implant; observe its transparency. (**d**) Histological section: the absence of a real biointegration leads to the detachment of the PEA sheet from the surrounding stroma. (**e**) A high implant extrusion rate was observed

Intrastromal Stem Cell Implant Along Decellularized Corneal Stroma

As we pointed out before, stromal synthetic substitutes have important limitations, and the isolated cellular therapy, although having promising results, does not seem good enough to rehabilitate completely a weak and thin cornea. Therefore, in these cases, it would be necessary to add a scaffold in order to enhance its therapeutic properties.

Over the past years, multiple methods of corneal decellularization have been developed, which provide a corneal acellular extracellular matrix [26]. These acellular tissues have been of great interest lately because they provide the most physiological environment possible to allow the growth and differentiation of stem cells into functional keratocytes while providing an immediate anatomical improvement with a theoretical absence of rejection risk by eliminating any antigenic cellular component. The components of extracellular matrix are pretty much conserved between different animal species, the reason why they are well tolerated even in xenogeneic scenarios without generating any inflammatory response.

As we have discussed, keratocytes are essential not only for the proper corneal stroma remodeling but also for a normal epithelial physiology [3]. This points out the importance of transplanting a cellular substitute along an acellular structural support to ensure a long-term corneal transparency through an adequate maintenance of the corneal homeostasis.

To our knowledge, all attempts to recolonize these decellularized stromal grafts have used corneal cells [27–29], but as we have mentioned, these cells have important limitations which complicate their use in clinical practice, hence the efforts to find an ideal extraocular source of autologous stem cells.

In our previous experimental study, we showed a perfect in vivo biointegration of decellularized human corneal stroma sheets with and without subsequent recellularization of human ADASCs, implanted inside the rabbit corneal stroma (Fig. 5), without any inflammatory response despite being a xenogeneic transplant [30].

We also showed in vivo stem cell differentiation into functional adult keratocytes inside these grafts, achieving a proper tissue function.

Through this transplant model, the advantages of corneal cell therapy would be obtained, while corneal anatomy is regenerated more efficiently in weakened corneas, without theoretical risk of rejection because the model allows to transform an allogeneic donor tissue into an autologous one.

Our research team recently published the first clinical essay in humans using decellularized tissue for the rehabilitation of the corneal stroma [31, 32]. In this study, we implanted inside intrastromal pockets dissected with femtosecond laser at half the corneal thickness measured by OCT decellularized human corneal stromal lenticules (120-micron-thick and 9-mm-diameter lenticules) (Video 2) with and without subsequent recellularization with autologous ADASCs of patients with terminal keratoconus [31, 32]. We could demonstrate a moderate but statistically significant improvement of all visual parameters (two lines of vision approximately),

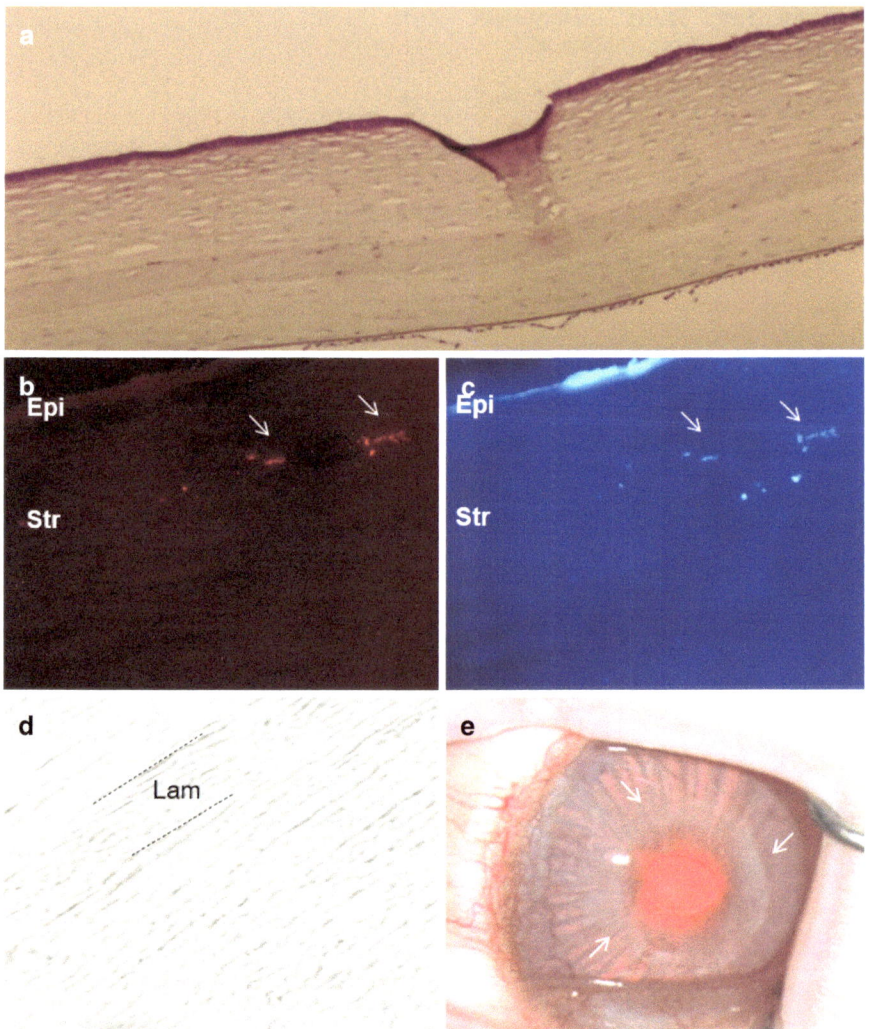

Fig. 5 Transplant of decellularized human corneal stroma with subsequent recellularization with human ADASCs inside rabbit stroma. (**a**) Hematoxylin-eosin: observe the perfect tissue biointegration (hypocellular strip of extracellular matrix) in absence of any inflammatory response. (**b**) Cellular survival at 3 months. (**c**) Cellular expression of human keratocan, specific marker of keratocyte differentiation. (**d**) Phase-contrast image showing a morphologically intact stroma. (**e**) Complete recovery of corneal transparency after transplant

with a reduction of refractive sphere, anterior keratometric flattening (Fig. 6f), and an improvement in corneal aberrometry, especially spherical aberration [31, 32]. After 3 months of observation, none of the patients developed any scarring or

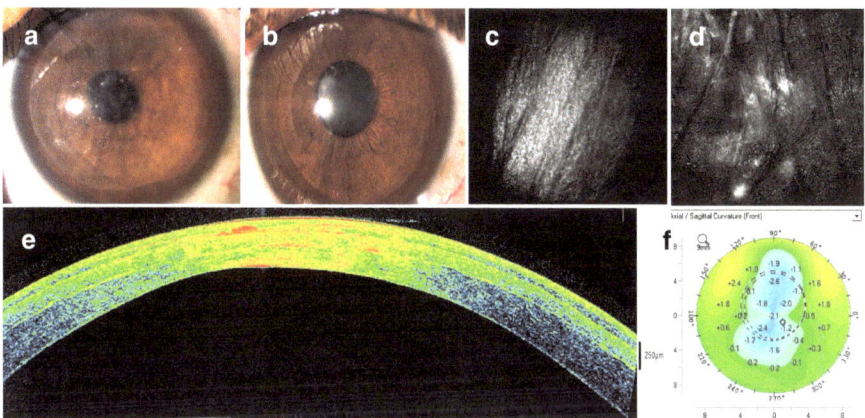

Fig. 6 Stromal scaffold with human decellularized corneal stroma with or without recellularization with human autologous ADASC. (**a**, **b**) Slit lamp images at 1 week (**a**) and 3 months (**b**) after implant. Observe the full recovery of corneal transparency. (**c**) Confocal microscopy of the implanted sheet showing a complete acellular pattern 3 months post-op. (**d**) First signs of recellularization of the sheet 12 months after surgery (images of a 100 × 100 μm area). (**e**) Anterior segment OCT 1 year after implant. Observe the perfect integration of the tissue and the restoration of corneal thickness. (**f**) Topographic changes between pre-op and 1 year post-op. Observe the central keratometric flattening

clinically significant haze (Fig. 6a, b), and all pachymetry parameters improved on average 120 microns, as expected, restoring the anatomy of these corneas with severe ectatic disease (Fig. 6e). On the other hand, we could not demonstrate any clinical differences between patients implanted with decellularized and recellularized sheets with autologous ADASCs, although the subsequent recellularization by host keratocytes of in vivo sheets was greater in those who received ADASCs with the implant (Fig. 6c, d) [31, 32].

Intracameral or Intravenous Stem Cell Injection

Demirayak reported that MSCs re-suspended in saline solution (PBS) and injected into the anterior chamber after a corneal penetrating trauma in a mouse model were capable of colonizing the corneal stroma and enhance the expression of keratocytic markers like keratocan as well as the keratocytic stromal density [33]. However, the possible clinical application of this model is questionable due to the possible effect of intracameral cellular injection of stem cells on the crystalline epithelium and the iridotrabecular angle, with potential obstruction of the trabeculum.

Intravenous injection of MSCs in recipient mice of an allogeneic cornea transplant was able to induce colonization of the transplanted cornea and conjunctiva of the recipient eye by MSCs, reducing associated immunity and improving graft survival [34].

Yun et al. reported similar findings after intravenous injection of MSCs derived from iPSC and BM-MSC after corneal caustications in the animal model, observing less inflammation and scarring than controls [35]. However, our group has not been able to confirm these results in the rabbit model, obtaining in contrast a lower survival of the transplanted graft compared to controls not treated systemically with MSC [36].

In conclusion, the regenerative and cellular therapy of the corneal stroma needs more investigation for its clinical use, since its real benefits are still to be defined, as well as the relevance of several of the clinical findings observed.

However, after multiple animal experimentation studies in recent years reporting very encouraging results, some research teams have made the leap to clinical trials in humans that will end up validating these new treatment modalities, so that in a few years, they can be either used in clinical practice or they will remain as a scientific curiosity.

Bibliography

1. De Miguel MP, Casaroli-Marano RP, Nieto-Nicolau N, Martínez-Conesa EM, Alió del Barrio JL, Alió JL, Fuentes S, Arnalich-Montiel F. Frontiers in regenerative medicine for cornea and ocular surface. In: Rahman AU, Anjum S, Bentham ED, editors. Frontiers in stem cell and regenerative medicine research; 2015. ISBN: 978-1-60805-995-9. Chapter 2. p. 92–138.
2. Carlson EC, Liu CY, Chikama T, et al. Keratocan, a cornea-specific keratan sulfate proteoglycan, is regulated by lumican. J Biol Chem. 2005;280:25541–7.
3. Wilson SE, Liu JJ, Mohan RR. Stromal-epithelial interactions in the cornea. Prog Retin Eye Res. 1999;18:293–309.
4. Du Y, Funderburgh ML, Mann MM, SundarRaj N, Funderburgh JL. Multipotent stem cells in human corneal stroma. Stem Cells. 2005;23:1266–75.
5. Ruberti JW, Zieske JD. Prelude to corneal tissue engineering – gaining control of collagen organization. Prog Retin Eye Res. 2008;27:549–77.
6. Takahashi K, Yamanaka S. Induction of pluripotent stem cells from mouse embryonic and adult fibroblast cultures by defined factors. Cell. 2006;126:663–76.
7. Harkin DG, Foyn L, Bray LJ, Sutherland AJ, Li FJ, Cronin BG. Concise reviews: can mesenchymal stromal cells differentiate into corneal cells? A systematic review of published data. Stem Cells. 2015;33:785–91.
8. Yao L, Bai H. Review: Mesenchymal stem cells and corneal reconstruction. Mol Vis. 2013;19:2237–43.
9. Caplan AI. Mesenchymal stem cells: time to change the name! Stem Cells Transl Med. 2017;6:1445–51.
10. Jiang Z, Liu G, Meng F, Wang W, Hao P, Xiang Y, et al. Paracrine effects of mesenchymal stem cells on the activation of keratocytes. Br J Ophthalmol. 2017;101:1583–90.
11. Di G, Du X, Qi X, Zhao X, Duan H, Li S, et al. Mesenchymal stem cells promote diabetic corneal epithelial wound healing through TSG-6-dependent stem cell activation and macrophage switch. Invest Ophthalmol Vis Sci. 2017;58(10):4344–54.
12. Agorogiannis GI, Alexaki VI, Castana O, Kymionis GD. Topical application of autologous adipose-derived mesenchymal stem cells (MSCs) for persistent sterile corneal epithelial defect. Graefes Arch Clin Exp Ophthalmol. 2012;250(3):455–7.

13. Basu S, Hertsenberg AJ, Funderburgh ML, Burrow MK, Mann MM, Du Y, et al. Human limbal biopsy-derived stromal stem cells prevent corneal scarring. Sci Transl Med. 2014;6(266):266ra172.
14. Basu S. Limbal stromal stem cell therapy for acute and chronic superficial corneal pathologies: early clinical outcomes with the Funderburgh technique. Oral presentation at The Association for Research in Vision and Ophthalmology (ARVO) Annual meeting; 2017; Baltimore (USA).
15. Arnalich-Montiel F, Pastor S, Blazquez-Martinez A, et al. Adipose-derived stem cells are a source for cell therapy of the corneal stroma. Stem Cells. 2008;26:570–9.
16. Du Y, Carlson EC, Funderburgh ML, et al. Stem cell therapy restores transparency to defective murine corneas. Stem Cells. 2009;27:1635–42.
17. Liu H, Zhang J, Liu CY, et al. Cell therapy of congenital corneal diseases with umbilical mesenchymal stem cells: lumican null mice. PLoS One. 2010;5:e10707.
18. Thomas VJCB, Kao WW. Transplantation of human umbilical mesenchymal stem cells cures the corneal defects of Mucopolysaccharidosis VII mice. Stem Cells. 2013;
19. Alió del Barrio JL, El Zarif M, de Miguel MP, et al. Cellular therapy with human autologous adipose-derived adult stem cells for advanced keratoconus. Cornea. 2017;36:952–60.
20. Espandar L, Bunnell B, Wang GY, et al. Adipose-derived stem cells on hyaluronic acid-derived scaffold: a new horizon in bioengineered cornea. Arch Ophthalmol. 2012;130:202–8.
21. Ma XY, Bao HJ, Cui L, Zou J. The graft of autologous adipose-derived stem cells in the corneal stromal after mechanic damage. PLoS One. 2013;8:e76103.
22. De Miguel MP, Alio JL, Arnalich-Montiel F, et al. Cornea and ocular surface treatment. Curr Stem Cell Res Ther. 2010;5:195–204.
23. Hu X, Lui W, Cui L, Wang M, Cao Y. Tissue engineering of nearly transparent corneal stroma. Tissue Eng. 2005;11:1710–7.
24. Mimura T, Amano S, Yokoo S, et al. Tissue engineering of corneal stroma with rabbit fibroblast precursors and gelatin hydrogels. Mol Vis. 2008;14:1819–28.
25. Alió Del Barrio JL, Chiesa M, Gallego Ferrer G, et al. Biointegration of corneal macroporous membranes based on poly(ethyl acrylate) copolymers in an experimental animal model. J Biomed Mater Res A. 2015;103:1106–18.
26. Lynch AP, Ahearne M. Strategies for developing decellularized corneal scaffolds. Exp Eye Res. 2013;108:42–7.
27. Choi JS, Williams JK, Greven M, et al. Bioengineering endothelialized neo-corneas using donor-derived corneal endothelial cells and decellularized corneal stroma. Biomaterials. 2010;31:6738–45.
28. Shafiq MA, Gemeinhart RA, Yue BY, Djalilian AR. Decellularized human cornea for reconstructing the corneal epithelium and anterior stroma. Tissue Eng Part C Methods. 2012;18:340–8.
29. Gonzalez-Andrades M, de la Cruz CJ, Ionescu AM, et al. Generation of bioengineered corneas with decellularized xenografts and human keratocytes. Invest Ophthalmol Vis Sci. 2011;52:215–22.
30. Alió del Barrio JL, Chiesa M, Garagorri N, et al. Acellular human corneal matrix sheets seeded with human adipose-derived mesenchymal stem cells integrate functionally in an experimental animal model. Exp Eye Res. 2015;132C:91–100.
31. Alió Del Barrio JL, El Zarif M, Azaar A, et al. Corneal stroma enhancement with decellularized stromal laminas with or without stem cell recellularization for advanced keratoconus. Am J Ophthalmol. 2018;186:47–58.
32. Alió JL, Alió Del Barrio JL, El Zarif M, et al. Regenerative medicine of the corneal stroma for advanced keratoconus: one year outcomes. Am J Ophthalmol 2019; [Accepted].
33. Demirayak B, Yüksel N, Çelik OS, et al. Effect of bone marrow and adipose tissue-derived mesenchymal stem cells on the natural course of corneal scarring after penetrating injury. Exp Eye Res. 2016;151:227–35.

34. Omoto M, Katikireddy KR, Rezazadeh A, Dohlman TH, Chauhan SK. Mesenchymal stem cells home to inflamed ocular surface and suppress allosensitization in corneal transplantation. Invest Ophthalmol Vis Sci. 2014;55:6631–8.
35. Yun YI, Park SY, Lee HJ, et al. Comparison of the anti-inflammatory effects of induced pluripotent stem cell-derived and bone marrow-derived mesenchymal stromal cells in a murine model of corneal injury. Cytotherapy. 2017;19:28–35.
36. Fuentes-Julián S, Arnalich-Montiel F, Jaumandreu L, et al. Adipose-derived mesenchymal stem cell administration does not improve corneal graft survival outcome. PLoS One. 2015;10:e0117945.

Corneal Remodeling: A New Alternative Technique to Treat Corneal Ectasia

César Carriazo and María José Cosentino

Introduction

In keratoconus, the poor visual acuity is due to irregular astigmatism of the anterior curvature of the cornea. Nowadays, the surgical management of keratoconus is based on three main pillars: *corneal cross-linking* (a technique which strengthens the anterior corneal stroma and makes the progression of keratoconus decrease), *intracorneal rings* (which base their mechanism on a calculated deformation of a corneal area to compensate the deformation caused by keratoconus), and *keratoplasties* (which structurally replace the weakened corneal tissue).

We propose an alternative treatment which attempts to flatten the cornea and give it its original shape. This is carried out by resecting a peripheral portion of the cornea and suturing resected edges. This is a surgical procedure which consists of a corneal stretching and is calculated for each patient. Even though we worked with laser excimer on our first patients (2014) by using protective masks to produce the size and shape of the wanted resection, we had to use femtosecond laser because the excimer laser is dependent on masks to produce the resections and the customized treatment for each patient restricts the use of such technology a lot.

Electronic Supplementary Material The online version of this chapter (https.//doi.org/10.1007/978-3-030-66143-4_10) contains supplementary material, which is available to authorized users.

C. Carriazo
Clínica Carriazo, Universidad del Norte, Barranquilla, Colombia

M. J. Cosentino (✉)
Instituto de la Vision, Universidad de Buenos Aires, Buenos Aires, Argentina

© Springer Nature Switzerland AG 2021
C. Carriazo, M. J. Cosentino (eds.), *New Frontiers for the Treatment of Keratoconus*, https://doi.org/10.1007/978-3-030-66143-4_10

New Concepts on Corneal Biomechanics

Stromal Volume and Redistribution

Thin corneas have better visual acuity than the thick ones, while the same symmetric conditions in their meridians are kept. This means the thinner the passage of light through the same structure is, the less alteration it suffers (refraction and diffraction) [1]. Therefore, corneal thinning in keratoconus per se does not generate poor visual acuity; it is the irregular astigmatism in the said pathology that causes high corneal aberrations which really produce the poor visual acuity.

We have observed in keratoconus that corneal stroma is not lost, but it is redistributed within the cornea, keeping its initial volume [2]. When the corneal stroma is redistributed, the thickness of the corneal stroma decreases at the expense of the steepening of the cornea. This means that the corneal volume of the total stroma of a healthy cornea is very similar to the one that has been rubbed and then has developed keratoconus.

A step forward would be to quantify the corneal epithelium when it produces compensatory changes in the zone of larger thinning; so we search for a larger regularity of the corneal surface [3].

Arc

In corneal topography, we make reference to radii (in millimeters) or keratometries (corneal radius turned into diopters), and we also refer to multiple radii.

Why do we refer to multiple radii? Because the cornea is not a sphere: it is an aspheric shell. For this reason, we have to measure multiple zones of the cornea, and we have to obtain the value of each of the said zones. Also, we have to give them a color according to the scale so as to produce topographic maps in order to help us understand the corneal morphology.

Due to the current topographies, these do not allow us to properly understand what happens in the whole cornea since they individually make their analysis in each reading point. Elevation topographies provide us with more information about biomechanical behavior. However, they are limited to give information from best fit sphere or a toric fit (toric and elliptic fit) which restrict their comparison and understanding.

Due to the abovementioned limitations and for a greater understanding of a pre- and postoperative keratoconic cornea, we want to introduce this new concept of "corneal arc." In order to understand its meaning better, the "corneal arc" is the distance in millimeters or microns which exits between limbo and limbo, follows the corneal curvature, and passes through the corneal center in its different meridians.

Therefore, we can say that in keratoconus, the corneal arcs gradually increase on account of the frequent rub of the cornea (allergies in most cases) or genetic alteration of the hardness of the stroma per se (genetic keratoconus).

As the corneal arc increases, the corneal structure becomes weaker; such increase is due to the corneal thickness decrease (redistribution of the stroma).

Corneal Remodeling

Knowing the "corneal volume" which was used by these corneas to increase their arcs and calculating the relation between "volume and arc," we calculated the volume which should be removed from this cornea to decrease its arcs so as to stretch and flatten the cornea.

When we resect the peripheral corneal tissue and suture its edges, a corneal stretching, which increases the corneal tension, is produced. As a result, we obtain a shortening of its arcs, as a consequence, a corneal flattening, which means, in topography terminology, there is an average increase of the radii of the corneal meridians (see Surgical Procedure).

It is important to make clear that the shortening of the radius of a sphere increases its curvature but the shortening of an arc in which the starting and finishing point remain unchanged (the limbo in the case of the cornea) decreases its curvature, which means the cornea is flattened. Based on this concept, we would be facing a new "corneal arc law": if the peripheral tissue is added to stretch the corneal arc, the cornea is steeped, and if the tissue is resected by shortening the corneal arc, the cornea is flattened.

Furthermore, a loose rope which is not stretched is either weak or flimsy, but when we stretch it, we achieve to increase its stiffness. A clear example of this is a tightrope walker who needs a tight rope to be able to walk on it. The said stiffness provides him with the necessary condition to walk on it.

This concept helps us understand what happens in the cornea with this new surgical technique: we increase the corneal tension and thus its rigidity. So, we can conclude that when we stretch the cornea (corneal remodeling), a corneal flattening is produced, and at the same time, this tension increases the corneal strength.

We not only have the cross-linking as a new additional alternative to increase even more its strength but we also have the abovementioned techniques. So, we can say that we have solved the keratoconus problem, its weakness, and the asymmetric steepening of the cornea.

It is not necessary to correct the thinning in keratoconus since thin corneas are shown to see well without any high-order optical aberrations [4]. The corneal thickness, therefore, is not necessary to be increased as long as the corneal anterior surface is regular and in its function as happens in this technique.

It is possible that such corneal stiffness produced by **Corneal Remodeling** technique, together with clear indications of not rubbing, is enough to give patients confidence. However, before confirming this, we are using cross-linking at 1.5 years since we performed **Corneal Remodeling** with a very good stability almost 6 years of follow-up.

Preoperative Exams

- Complete refractive exam
- Corneal topography and tomography
- Biometry
- Interferometry or power lens measurements
- Corneal OCT
- Aberrometry
- Endothelial cell count

Refraction Exam

The refractive dysfunction of the patient, the keratometries, the axis of astigmatism, and the far and near best visual acuity obtained allow us to have an idea about the stage of keratoconus we are going to face. Also, we will classify and perform the surgical plan for the said patient taking into account the other preoperative exams.

Each keratoconic eye is treated in a different way due to the fact such technique tries to correct not only the irregular astigmatism of keratoconus but the refractive dysfunction of the whole eye as well.

We state that because it is frequent to associate keratoconus with other dysfunctions inherent to the eye shape and size and its keratometric relation. The most frequent one is the myopia and astigmatism. This means that the same topographic pattern of keratoconus may need a thoroughly different treatment which depends on other variables such as biometry, corneal diameter, and power of lens.

Corneal Topography and Tomography

The topographic descriptions of keratoconus may be obtained by different technologies. We are currently using the elevation corneal tomography, Placido's ring topography, and the OCT. The most significant information to be obtained about these technologies is the anterior topographic pattern, keratometry, pachymetry, white-to-white information, anterior chamber depth measurement, and corneal volume and arc.

(a) *Anterior topographic pattern:* This allows us to classify the stage of keratoconus.

1. Central pattern whose apex is in the central millimeter of the cornea
2. Inferior pattern whose apex is more than 1 mm from the corneal center
3. Temporal pattern whose apex is more than 1 mm from the corneal center
4. Nasal pattern whose apex is more than 1 mm from the corneal center
5. Inferior and temporal pattern (the most frequent) whose apex is in the temporal inferior area of the cornea

(b) *Keratometry*

This is a very difficult value to be manually found due to the fact we find multiple keratometry values within the optical zone. This is the reason why we use the topographic average value:

- K: central value
- CIM: stages of irregularity
- TKM: toric keratometry
- I–S: superior–inferior difference
- CEI: measures corneal centering
- ACP: measures the average corneal power
- SDP: measures the standard power deviation
- DSI: compares one different area
- OSI: compares two opposite areas
- CSI: Compares an area with a sector which is closed
- IAI: measures the irregular astigmatism
- AA: a comparison between the analyzed area and the total of the topography
- SAI: a surface symmetry
- SRI: stages of irregular surface

(c) *Pachymetry map:* This is the necessary value to determine the depth of the resection. We normally suggest using a depth between 80 and 90% of the lower thickness found in the pachymetry map at an 8 mm diameter.

(d) *White-to-white:* this is the necessary value to estimate the appropriate calculation of the planned resection. Flattening an 11 mm cornea does not have the same effect as flattening a 13 mm cornea. The calculation is automatically carried out by the software, and its incorporation in the calculation of the resection was recommended by Dr. David Flikier.

(e) *Anterior chamber:* On one hand, even though the anterior chamber of the patients with keratoconus is usually deep, it is necessary to take this into account because in deep resections, the anterior chamber angle might be affected. On the other hand, decreasing the anterior chamber depth slightly contributes to compensating the myopia of the patient.

(f) *Corneal volume:* This is a numerical calculation variable which helps us know the amount of tissue to be resected.

(g) *Corneal arc:* This is a new concept we are developing and is not available in the current technologies.

Biometry

This is necessary to calculate expected K since our calculation is focused on correcting not only the refractive dysfunction of the eye but the irregular astigmatism induced by the ectasia as well.

Interferometry or Lens Power Measurement

Nowadays, it is statistically assumed, but it will be able to be measured very soon by new technologies. This technology is necessary to determine the expected K for each patient.

OCT

This tool is useful not only to show the behavior of the stroma thickness and the corneal epithelium but to determine the resection depth as well. In this way, we will be able to understand the postoperative biomechanics of these patients.

Aberrometry

This exam is very useful for us to explain the different types of corrected visual acuity these cases usually develop; and then, we may very well be able to provide effective follow-up.

Endothelial Cell Count

This exam is important to show the reliability of such surgical technique, since we approach the endothelial layer within the resection area.

Surgical Planning

The resection calculation is made by a software (Carriazo/Cosentino/Flikier) which is completed with different variables suggested by the same software [5, 6].

The software based on the above information recommends a treatment which can be modified or adapted by the doctor according to the target he wants for each patient.

The modifiable variants of the software are:

Geometric Figure (See *Fig. 1*)

(a) Ring symmetry
(b) Complete crescentic keratectomy (360 degrees)
(c) Incomplete crescentic keratectomy (less than 360 degrees)
(d) Decreasing–crescentic (ellipsoid)

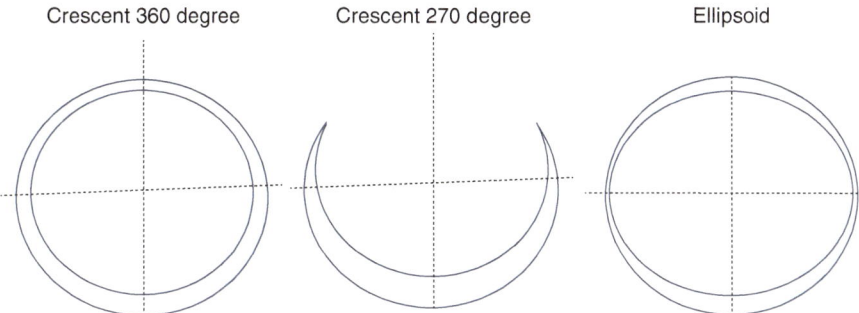

Fig. 1 Diagram of the geometric figures of the keratectomies

Gap

This variable depends on the corneal flattening stage and the amount of reduction of the anterior chamber depth (ACD). The reduction of anterior chamber affects the postoperative biometry and, therefore, contributes to reducing the preoperative myopia.

Resection Depth

We suggest not creating a corneal perforation in order to work in a more controlled way and not to have an abrupt loss of aqueous humor and anterior chamber collapse which endangers the inner structures of the eye.

Our study has based its results on depths between 80 and 90% of the thinnest point which is 8 mm from the cornea. This is calculated by the pachymetric data which the elevation topographers or the preoperative OCT provide, and it can be adjusted, if necessary, during the procedure following the intraoperative OCT.

Optical Zone

In order to have standardization and a better understanding of the corneal biomechanics, so far we have only worked with an optical zone of an outer 8 mm diameter, and the resections are performed within this optical zone.

Despite the fact the optical zone defined by default is 8 mm, in the future, we will be able to go into reducing such zone either to get a better correction or increase it to be able to treat further peripheral degenerations such as keratoglobus or keratotorus.

Centering

The geometrically selected figure is centered according to the patient's pupil or to the limbo in the same cases.

Surgical Procedure

When we started developing this technique, we used SCHWIND AMARIS excimer laser (Eye-Tech-Solutions, Germany) with a platform developed for us so as to perform ring peripherical ablations, and we used masks with different openings and figures to make such surgery. However, its limitations on the planning and customization for each patient made us migrate to femtosecond technology which is the one we are currently working and we recommend and is detailed below.

We have developed a software together with Ziemer (Ziemer Group, Switzerland) to perform such **corneal remodeling** technique by using the platform of its Z8 femtosecond laser version.

Under topic anesthesia and a light sedation, we place sterile fields and use different types of speculum to have the patient's cornea properly exposed. We place the suction ring which is in the disposable package used by Ziemer to keep the eye fixed. The software will allow us to proceed to the next step unless a proper suction is obtained. Once this proper suction is obtained, the arm and mobile head of the laser are connected with the suction ring.

When the abovementioned step is done, an image of the corneal centering and OCT will appear on the screen. At this moment, one has the option to choose the depth of the resection one wishes to use in each case by following the intraoperative OCT. The screen also shows the above geometrically selected figure with the thickness of the gap for every quadrant.

Moreover, the option of the centering of the resection is simultaneously shown on the screen. This shows some arrows in four different directions developed for this purpose. By using such arrows, the geometrically selected figure is properly centered according to the patient's pupil and in some cases to the limbo.

As Fig. 2 shows, once the desired parameters are selected, the laser equipment calculates the procedure for 90 seconds approximately. In this way, the procedure is activated (at this moment, the screen shows the progression of the said step).

When the procedure is finished, the suction is automatically set off, and then, the complex head ring of the laser is removed from the eye. Then, a temporary paracentesis is performed under surgical microscope, and the aqueous humor is drained to put less intraocular pressure in the AC, which allows an easy corneal suture.

The outer and inner gap of the resection is verified by using a fine spatula and by checking the joint bridges do not remain since they may be left by using femtosecond technology.

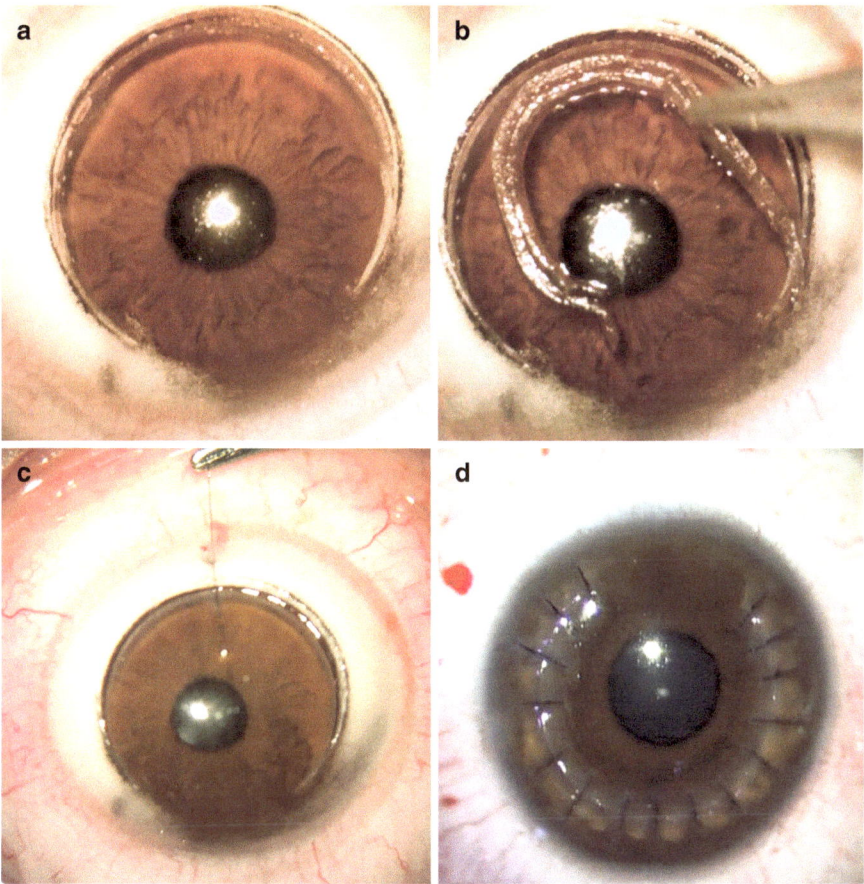

Fig. 2 Surgical technique steps. (**a**) Crescentic keratectomy. (**b**) Removal of the resection. (**c**) Suture. (**d**) Complete suture

Once this is verified by using a 0.12 tong, the corneal tissue is removed by the laser. When the resection is at 360 degrees, 24 nylon 10/0 separated stitches are used to close the edges, and when the resection is lower than 360 degrees, a smaller number of stitches are used. By doing so, we attempt to face the corneal opposing edges in a perfect way.

Even though the number of sutures may be less, we have observed that using this number does not allow openings between sutures (fish-mouth-shaped opening). A large number of sutures allow removing them before according to the postoperative astigmatism which is observed. Nevertheless, we are currently developing alternatives which allow us to reduce the number of sutures with the same astigmatic control.

Once the suture is finished, we prescribe tobramycin combined with dexamethasone ophthalmologic ointment followed by ocular occlusion for 24 hours. Then

Fig. 3 Postoperative slit
lamp examiination at 1
year of Corneal
Remodeling technique

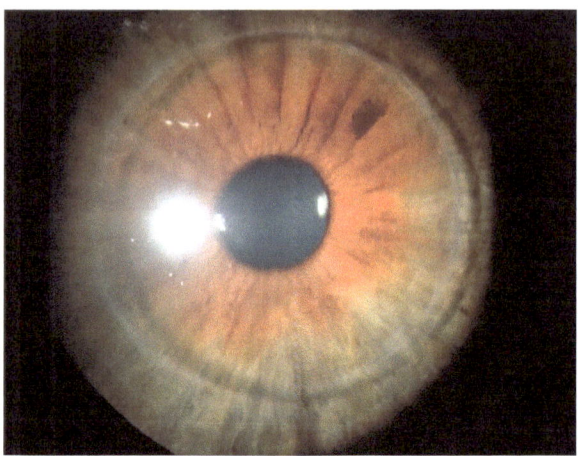

moxifloxacin combined with dexamethasone drop is prescribed every 6 hours for 10 days and artificial tear drops every 8 hours for 3 months. Once the 10 days of antibiotic with corticosteroid is completed, we continue with fluorometholone every 8 hours for 1 month.

In the immediate period, every loose suture must be removed, which is normally identified when the mucus is accumulated and this becomes stained with fluorescein. The sutures are gradually removed after about the fourth month; we are guided by the patient's refraction and corneal topography. For people aged over 40 years, we start removing the sutures at the 6th month, and at 1-year surgery, approximately, the whole sutures have been removed. Figure 3 shows a clear postoperative with all the sutures removed.

Complementary Procedures

In order to think about performing a complementary refractive surgery, we wait for a year without sutures and when we see stability which means having two similar refractive controls separated by 6 months; at this stage, we consider performing a complementary surgery.

Due to the fact we perform a customized resection for each patient, the residual refractive errors are low and can be generally corrected by surface ablation techniques. We perform the said procedure together with corneal cross-linking for the time being. Also, we program a residual target of −0.5 diopters to compensate the flattening caused by the latter.

The maximum follow-up time we have is 6 years, and the stability observed has been from good to excellent. It should be pointed out that these patients are very conscious of not rubbing their eyes, which, in our opinion, is one of the most important aspects to achieve refractive stability in such cases.

Analysis of the Cases

After analyzing the first 125 cases, we have to emphasize the following concepts:

- In all the cases, we have observed the corneal flattening, which means the increase of the radius of corneal curvature.
- In all cases, we gained corrected visual acuity lines, with an average of almost three gained lines. None of the cases lost visual acuity lines.
- The uncorrected visual acuity has been superior to 20/40 in many cases without being the main purpose of such procedure.
- The sutures must not be early removed so as to control the desired refractive result. According to this, we have considered that shorter sutures and in greater number may generate even more refractive predictability.
- In all the cases, there was a coma reduction in particular, and there was a high-order aberration (HOA) reduction in general.
- A significant refractive phenomenon is the reduction of the anterior chamber depth. The said anterior chamber depth in this sequence of cases was reduced to an average close to 0.400 mm.
- The endothelial cell count showed an endothelial cell loss lower than 5% after the first postoperative year.
- In the slit lamp exam, a crescentic arc of wound healing with an optical zone of 8 mm appears. Due to the wound healing and stiffness itself, this zone has a behavior which can well be described as a new "biomechanical limbo" because of the limbic strengthening which this wound healing produces [7–28].

Last Considerations

Figures 4, 5, 6, and 7 show the obtained refractive results at almost 6-year follow-up. It is important to consolidate some ideas for a better understanding of this new concept. The progression of keratoconus is accompanied by the increase of the anterior chamber by means of the increase of posterior corneal curvature, corneal thinning, and progressive corneal steepening.

The crescentic or annular keratectomy technique with laser – **corneal remodeling** – is a safe procedure which produces corneal flattening, reduces anterior chamber depth, reduces optical aberrations, and offers a wide optical zone which allows the performance of complementary refractive techniques. The studies made by a computer simulation have let us not only ratify the obtained clinical results but lead us to the surgical nomogram bases as well.

Nearly 5 years of the first performed cases, we introduce the **corneal remodeling** (Carriazo C., Cosentino, MJ. "A novel corneal remodeling technique for the management of keratoconus." J Refract Surg 2017; 33 (12): 854 and "Long-Term Outcomes for a New Surgical technique for Corneal Remodeling in Cornea Ectasia."

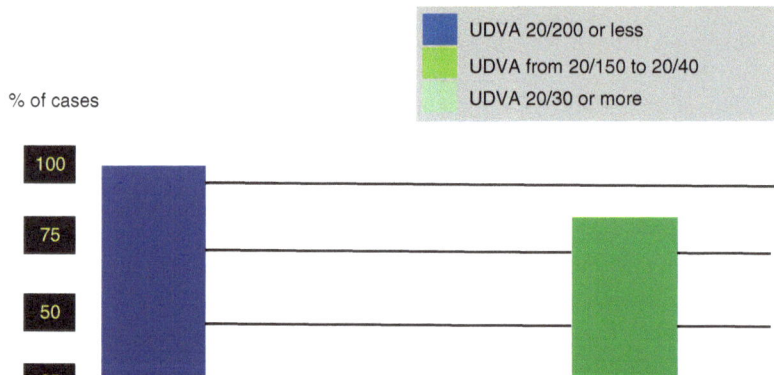

Fig. 4 Uncorrected distance visual acuity

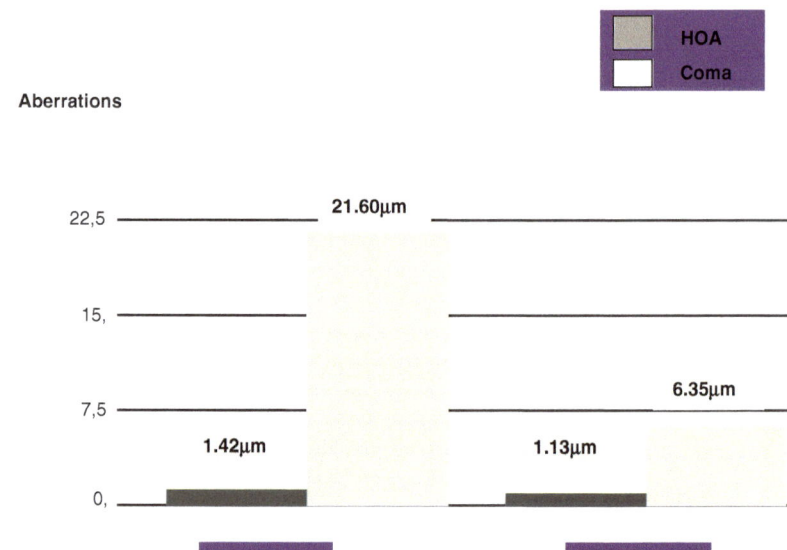

Fig. 5 High-order aberrations

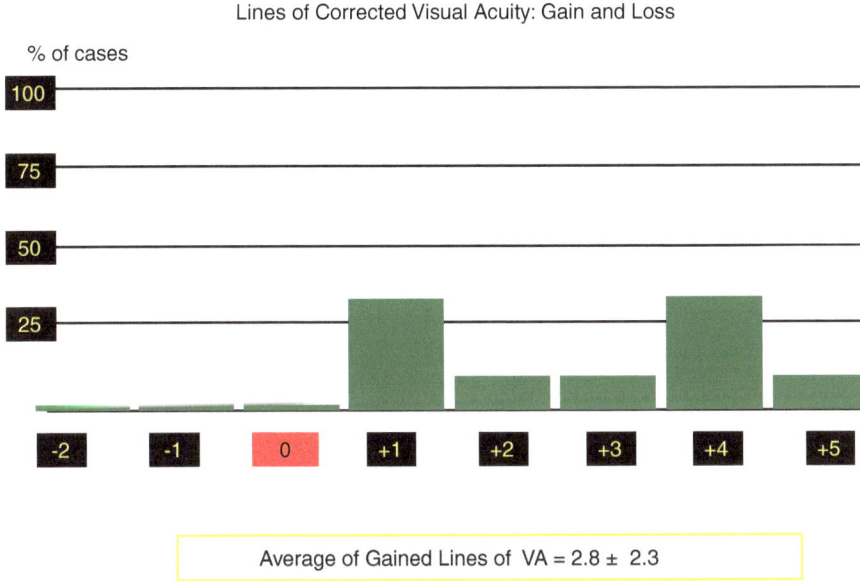

Fig. 6 Gained and lost lines of visual acuity

Changes @ Steepest Meridian

	Pre-Op	Post-Op
Steepest meridian (Degree)	67.22	114.16

Fig. 7 Astigmatism change

J Refract Surg 2019;35 (4): 261–267) as a new surgical alternative in the management of keratoconus.

Different kinds of laser such as excimer and femtosecond and other lasers of different states may be used for the performance of this technique; we have preferred to develop this technique by using femtosecond laser. Different technologies of corneal analyses such as topographers, pachymetries, and OCT may be complementarily used for such purpose.

Due to the corneal stiffness produced by the corneal cross-linking, this might be considered a next step in the search for corneal stability. It would be expected that the association with corneal cross-linking treatment might give a greater corneal stability in the future [29, 30].

To sum up, we belive Corneal Remodeling (Video 1) represents a new approach to treat corneal ectasia; such technique allows us to reacquire the physiological lost profile in these types of corneas and enables us to perform complementary refractive corrections for an integral treatment of corneal ectasia.

References

1. Smith AM. Descartes's theory of light and refraction: a discourse on method. Am Philos Soc. 1987;
2. Cui J, Zhang X, Zhou WY, et al. Evaluation of corneal thickness and volume parameters of subclinical keratoconus using Pentacam system. Curr Eye Res. 2016;41(7):923–6.
3. Reinstein D, Archer TJ, Gobbe M. Corneal epithelial thickness profile in the diagnosis of keratoconus. Refract Surg. 2009;25(7):604–10.
4. Sasamoto M, Gonzalo M. Estudios del espesor corneal en pacientes de consulta general del IROJSU. Facultad de Medicina UNT. http://dspace.unitru.edu.pe/handle/UNITRU/533
5. Carriazo C, Cosentino MJ. A novel corneal remodeling technique for the treatment of keratoconus. J Refract Surg. 2017:155–8.
6. Carriazo C, Cosentino MJ. Corneal Remodeling assisted by femtosecond laser: long term outcomes. J Refract Surg 2019: Surgery. 2019;35(4):261–7.
7. Parker JS, van Dijk K, Melles GRJ. Treatment options for advanced keratoconus: a review. Surv Ophthalmol. 2015, Copyright © 2015 Elsevier Inc., pág. 22.
8. Sykakis E, Karim R, Evans JR, Bunce C, Amissah-Arthur KN, Patwary S, PJ MD. Corneal collagen cross-linking for treating keratoconus. Cochrane Library. 3
9. Wojcik KA, Blasiak J, Sza ik J, Sza ik JP. Role of biochemical factors in the pathogenesis of keratoconus. Acta Biochim Pol. 2014;61(1):55–62.
10. Zadnik, Karla y Lindsley, Kristina. s.l.: Cochrane Eyes and Vision Group. Intrastromal corneal ring segments for treating keratoconus. 2014, Vols. EBM Reviews – Cochrane Database of Systematic Reviews.
11. Alio JL, Vega-Estrada A, Esperanza S, Barraquer RI, Teus MA, Murta J. Intrastromal corneal ring segments: how successful is the surgical treatment of keratoconus? Middle East Afr J Ophthalmol. 2014;21(1):3–9.
12. Ganesh S, Shetty R, D'Souza S, Ramachandran S, Kurian M. Intrastromal corneal ring segments for management of keratoconus. Indian J Ophthal- mol. 2013;61(8):451–5.
13. Vega-Estrada A, Alio JL, Brenner LF, Javaloy J, Puche ABP, Barraquer RI, Teus MA, Murta J, Henriques J, Uceda-Montanes A. Outcome analysis of intracorneal ring segments for the treatment of keratoconus based on visual, refractive, and aberrometric impairment. Número 3, s.l. Am J Ophthalmol. 2013;Volúmen 155:575–584. e1.
14. McMonnies CW. Inflammation and keratoconus. Optom Vis Sci. 2015;92(2):35–41.
15. Maycock NJ, Marshall J. Genomics of corneal wound healing: a review of the literature. Acta Ophthalmol. 2014;92(3):e170–84.
16. Cheung IM, McGhee CN, Sherwin T. A new perspective on the pathobiology of keratoconus: interplay of stromal wound healing and reactive species-associated processes. Clin Exp Optom. 2013;96(2):188–96.
17. You J, Wen L, Roufas A, Madigan MC, Sutton G. Expression of SFRP family proteins in human keratoconus corneas. PLoS One. 2013;8(6):667–70.
18. Barbaro V, Di Iorio E, Ferrari S, Bisceglia L, Ruzza A, De Luca M, Pellegrini G. Expression of VSX1 in human corneal keratocytes during differentiation into myofibroblasts in response to wound healing. Invest Ophthalmol Vis Sci. 2006;47(12):5243–50.
19. Tuori AJ, Virtanen I, Aine E, Kalluri R, Miner JH, Uusitalo HM. The immuno- histochemical composition of corneal basement membrane in keratoconus. Curr Eye Res. 1997;16(8):792–801.
20. Zhou L, Yue BY, Twining SS, Sugar J, Feder RS. Expression of wound healing and stress-related proteins in keratoconus corneas. Curr Eye Res. 1996;15(11):1124–31.
21. Ezra DG, Hay-Smith G, Mearza A, Falcon MG. Corneal wedge excision in the treatment of high astigmatism after penetrating keratoplasty. Cornea. 2007;26(7):819–25.
22. Hoppenreijs VP, van Rij G, Beekhuis WH, Rijneveld WJ, Rinkel-van Driel E. Long-term results of corneal wedge resections for the correction of high astigmatism. Doc Ophthalmol. 1990;75(3–4):263–73.

23. Lugo M, Donnenfeld ED, Arentsen JJ. Corneal wedge resection for high astigmatism following penetrating keratoplasty. Ophthalmic Surg. 1987;18(9):650–3.
24. Durand L, Chahid B. Primary wedge resection of the cornea for keratoconus deformity. J Fr Opthalmol. 1993;16(11):626–719.
25. Erie JC. Corneal wound healing after photorefractive keratectomy: a 3-year confocal microscopy study. Trans Am Ophthalmol Soc. 2003;101:293–333.
26. Erie JC, McLaren JW, Hodge DO, Bourne WM. Recovery of corneal subbasal nerve density after PRK and LASIK. Am J Ophthalmol. 2005;140(6):1059–64.
27. Baldwin HC, Marshall J. Growth factors in corneal wound healing following refractive surgery: a review. Acta Ophthalmol Scand. 2002;80(3):238–47.
28. Fagerholm P. Wound healing after photorefractive keratectomy. J Cataract Refract Surg. 2000;26(3):432–47.
29. De Bernardo M, Capasso L, Lanza M, Tortori A, Iaccarino S, Cennamo M, et al. Long-term results of corneal collagen crosslinking for progressive keratoconus. J Optom. 2015;8(3):180–6.
30. Alhayek A, Lu PR. Corneal collagen crosslinking in keratoconus and other eye disease. Int J Ophthalmol. 2015;8(2):407–18.

Index

A
Aberrations, 103
Adipose derived adult stem cells, 111
Adipose human tissue, 111
Applanation lengths (AL), 10
Astigmatism, 2

B
Barraquer's law, 3

C
Centering, 130
Chronic Apical Distal and late Keratitis
    (CADLK), 80
Collagen cross-linking (CXL), 84
Cornea, 55–59
Corneal biomechanical index (CBI), 18
Corneal biomechanics, 4, 8
Corneal cross-linking (CXL), 56, 58, 59
Corneal remodeling, 125, 133, 135
    aberrometry, 128
    analyzing, 133
    arc, 124
    biometry, 127
    complementary procedures, 132
    corneal topography, 126, 127
    interferometry, 128

preoperative exams, 126
redistribution, 124
refraction exam, 126
stromal volume, 124
surgical planning, 128, 129
surgical procedure, 130–132
tomography, 126, 127
Corneal resistance factor (CRF), 8–9
Corneal topography, 8, 29, 32, 34, 37, 38, 99
Corneal transplant, 114
Corneal velocities (CVel), 10
Corrected distance visual acuity
    (CDVA), 86, 92
Corvis prototype-factor (CPF-1), 17
Crosslinking, 57–59

E
Ectatic corneal disease, 8, 18
Epithelial thickness, 28, 29
Excimer laser, 99, 100, 102, 103

G
Gross macroscopy, 49

H
Higher-order aberrations (HOAs), 84

© Springer Nature Switzerland AG 2021
C. Carriazo, M. J. Cosentino (eds.), *New Frontiers for the Treatment
of Keratoconus*, https://doi.org/10.1007/978-3-030-66143-4

I

Implantable collamer lens, keratoconus, 89, 90
Intracorneal rings segments (ICRS)
    anatomy
        apical diameter, 62, 63
        asymmetric segments, 69
        base, 62–64
        ends, 65
        external edge, 64
        inner edge, 65
        material, 62
        primary ectasias, 71
        thickness, 66, 67
    primary ectasias
        CADLK, 80
        patterns, 71
        stages, 72, 74, 75, 77–79
Irregular astigmatism, 99, 100, 103, 123, 124

K

Keratoconus, 1–4, 8, 42, 55, 56, 59, 83, 85, 99,
        100, 102–104, 106
    automated algorithm, 39, 40, 42
    clinical experience, 58, 59
    corneal epithelium, 34, 35
    corvis ST dynamic scheimpflug analyzer,
        9, 10, 14, 17, 18
    epithelial thickness, 29, 30, 32–35, 39
    histopathology, 49–53
    intergrated parameters, 18, 19
    light microscopy, 49
    limitations, 56, 57
    ocular response analyzer, 8, 9
    sensitivity, 27
    technical requirements, 56, 57
Keratocytes, 109, 110, 115–117, 119
Kic intraocular lens power calculation, 88

L

Light microscopy, 49

M

Manifest refractive spherical equivalent
    (MRSE), 86

N

Non-contact tonometry (NCT), 9

O

Ocular response analyzer (ORA), 8–10
Optical zone, 129

P

Phakic intraocular lenses (pIOLs),
    85–88, 93, 95
Phakic refractive lens (PRL), 85

R

Resection depth, 129
Rigid gas-permeable (RGP), 84

S

Sensitivity, 27
Software calculation, 103, 105
Stem cell implantation, 113, 115

T

Tissue engineering, 109, 110
    stem cells, 110–112
        therapeutic techniques, 112, 113, 115–117,
        119, 120
Tomographic-biomechanical index
    (TBI), 18, 21
Tomography, 28, 29, 43
Topography, 28, 32, 36, 84
Topography-assisted refraction, 74
Toric ICL (TICL), 89

U

Uncorrected distance visual acuity
    (UDVA), 91
US food and drug administration (FDA), 85

W

White-to-white (WTW), 88